Errata

Bowel care in older people
Research and practice

*Edited by Jonathan Potter, Christine Norton
and Alan Cottenden*

Acknowledgements

The Acknowledgements should have included thanks to
the Sir Halley Stewart Trust and **AgeCare** (formerly the Royal
Surgical Aid Society) for financial support towards the cost of
the workshop upon which this book is based.

Chapter 6, page 77

Laxative misuse. The expenditure of £43 billion quoted in the
first line under this heading should read £43 million.

List of participants

James Barrett *Consultant Physician in Geriatric Medicine and Rehabilitation, Clatterbridge Hospital, Wirral, Merseyside*

Alan Cottenden *Senior Lecturer, Department of Medical Physics, University College London*

Anton Emmanuel *Senior Lecturer and Consultant Gastroenterologist, St Mark's Hospital, London*

Mandy Fader *Lecturer, Department of Medicine, University College London; Continence Product Evaluation Network*

Jane Fenton *Clinical Nurse Specialist (Continence Promotion), North Staffs Combined Healthcare NHS Trust*

Danielle Harari *Senior Lecturer in Elderly Medicine, St Thomas' Hospital Elderly Care Unit, Guy's, King's and St Thomas' Hospital School of Medicine, London*

John Lennard-Jones *Emeritus Professor of Gastroenterology, Royal London Hospital Medical College, London*

James Malone-Lee *Professor of Medicine, University College Hospital, London*

Cath McGrother *Senior Lecturer in Epidemiology, University of Leicester; Lead, MRC Continence Programme*

Katherine Moore *Assistant Professor of Nursing, University of Alberta, Canada*

Linda Nazarko *Director, Nightingale Nursing Home, London; Visiting Senior Lecturer, South Bank University*

Christine Norton *Nurse Consultant (Bowel Control), St Mark's Hospital, North West London Hospitals NHS Trust, Harrow; Honorary Professor of Nursing, King's College, London*

Jonathan Potter *Consultant Geriatrician, Kent and Canterbury Hospital; Associate Director (Health Care of Older People), Clinical Effectiveness and Evaluation Unit, Royal College of Physicians, London*

Jolyon Rose *Executive Director, Incontact, London*

Paul Smith *Consultant Clinical Psychologist, Newcastle upon Tyne*

Graham Stokes *Consultant Clinical Psychologist, South Staffordshire Healthcare NHS Trust, Lichfield, Staffordshire; Consultant Director of Mental Health, BUPA Care Homes*

Caroline Vaizey *Consultant Colorectal Surgeon, University College Hospital, London*

Mandy Wells *Senior Nurse Specialist, St Pancras Hospital, London*

Helen White *Director, PromoCon, Cheetham, Manchester*

Bowel care in older people

Research and practice

Edited by

Jonathan Potter

Consultant Geriatrician, Kent and Canterbury Hospital;
Associate Director, Clinical Effectiveness and Evaluation Unit, Royal College of Physicians

Christine Norton

Nurse Consultant (Bowel Control), St Mark's Hospital, North West London Hospitals NHS
Trust; Honorary Professor of Nursing, King's College, London

Alan Cottenden

Senior Lecturer, Department of Medical Physics, University College London

2002

Clinical Effectiveness
& Evaluation Unit

ROYAL COLLEGE OF PHYSICIANS

The Clinical Effectiveness and Evaluation Unit (CEEU)

The Clinical Effectiveness and Evaluation Unit of the Royal College of Physicians concentrates on those issues that are at the centre of the national healthcare agenda, eg the National Service Frameworks in Cardiology, Care of Older People and Diabetes, and the Calman-Hine Cancer Framework, as a continuous programme of work rather than multiple one-off projects. Associate Directors, who are active clinicians in their field, lead the relevant programmes in conjunction with the Director. CEEU has expertise in the development of guidelines, the organising and reporting of multi-centre comparative audit to encourage guideline implementation, and studies on how the outcome of care can be measured reliably. All our work is collaborative with relevant specialist societies, patient groups and health service bodies such as the National Service Frameworks, National Institute for Clinical Excellence (NICE) and, in future, the Commission for Health Improvement (CHI). CEEU is self-financing with funding coming from government, charities and other organisations.

Royal College of Physicians of London
11 St Andrews Place, London NW1 4LE

Registered Charity No. 210508

Copyright © 2002 Royal College of Physicians of London

ISBN 1 86016 167 7

Cover design by Merriton Sharp

Typeset by Dan-Set Graphics, Telford, Shropshire

Printed in Great Britain by The Lavenham Press Ltd, Sudbury, Suffolk

Foreword

Faecal incontinence, unlike urinary incontinence, is not recognised as a major problem among ambulant community dwelling older people, though its impact can be devastating for those who suffer it. Minor degrees are probably endured in silence and go unreported to doctors, nurses or social workers. On the other hand, faecal incontinence is recognised as a major scourge of disabled institutionalised elderly people who live in residential homes and nursing homes. It is also a scourge for the staff who care for them.

Constipation, which is often associated with faecal incontinence, is almost certainly one of the most common symptoms perceived by people as they get older, often when the frequency of their bowel motions is well within what is regarded as normal.

Faecal incontinence, like other major problems in the medicine of old age, involves a multiplicity of contributing causes. These include biological ageing, diseases especially of the central nervous and gastro-intestinal systems and weight-bearing joints, psychiatric illness, long-term effects of childbirth, medications, changes in the pattern of daily living, nursing procedures – and even the design of buildings.

Despite the prevalence and wide-ranging associated effects of constipation and faecal incontinence, they have not hitherto appealed to clinical researchers as fruitful (or even feasible) fields of study. Yet common sense and such evidence as is available (expertly reviewed in the pages that follow) indicate a plethora of possible interventions to be evaluated and implemented. The sections entitled 'What we don't know' at the end of each chapter provide an extensive menu of research waiting to be undertaken. Some of these projects may be sufficiently short and self-contained to be carried out as a one-off by doctors or nurses in training. Others would provide a rolling research portfolio for a multidisciplinary team.

The report ends with an extensive series of practice guidance under 12 headings. Each of these sections could provide an audit session for staff training in nursing homes, primary care and hospital units.

This comprehensive report forms a landmark in relation to research and practice regarding bowel care for older people. It is highly commended, both for study and for serious action.

Professor John Brocklehurst
September 2002

v

Acknowledgements

We would like to thank all the participants for their time and interest in attending the workshop on bowel care in older people and for reviewing and commenting on the information presented. In particular we would like to thank the speakers for the additional trouble they took in reviewing the literature, presenting their findings and reviewing their texts submitted for publication.

We are grateful to Rob Grant of the Clinical Effectiveness and Evaluation Unit of the Royal College of Physicians, London, for his help in organising and ensuring the smooth running of the workshop.

The workshop was supported by grants from Norgine Ltd and from the Royal Surgical Aids Society.

Jonathan Potter
Christine Norton
Alan Cottenden

Contents

RESEARCH

PERSONAL PERSPECTIVES

APPENDIX 1

PRACTICE GUIDANCE

Glossary

Anal endosonography: ultrasound examination of the anal sphincter muscles.

Anorectal angle: the angle between the rectum and anus.

Anorectal incontinence: incontinence due to anorectal pathology or dysfunction.

Colectomy: surgical removal of the colon.

Constipation: infrequent or difficult bowel evacuation.

Defaecation: passing stool.

Dyschezia: difficulty with rectal evacuation.

Enteric nervous system: intrinsic nerve supply of the gut.

External anal sphincter: voluntary striated muscle component of the anal muscle ('back passage').

Faecal incontinence: loss of stool that is a social or hygienic problem.

Faecal loading/impaction/rectal loading: severe stasis of hard or soft stool in the colon and/or rectum.

Functional incontinence: incontinence due to functional (physical or mental) inability to use the toilet in a socially accepted manner.

Hirschsprung's disease: a congenital absence of nerves supplying the lowest portion of the rectum.

Impaction: *see* Faecal loading.

Incontinence: *see* Anorectal incontinence, Faecal incontinence, Functional incontinence, Overflow incontinence.

Internal anal sphincter: involuntary smooth muscle component of the anal muscle ('back passage').

Manual evacuation: emptying the rectum using a finger to extract stool.

Myenteric plexus: network of the enteric nervous system, the intrinsic nerve supply of the gut.

Obstructed defaecation: usually a failure of normal relaxation of the anal sphincter and pelvic floor muscles.

Overflow incontinence: (also sometimes termed 'spurious diarrhoea'): faecal incontinence secondary to faecal loading of the bowel.

Proctography/proctogram: x-ray study of the configuration of the rectum and anus, at rest and during straining and emptying.

Puborectalis muscles: the posterior portion of the pelvic floor muscles.

Pudendal nerve terminal motor latency: electrophysiological measurement of pudendal nerve conduction time.

Pudendal neuropathy: damage to the pudendal nerve which supplies the pelvic floor and sphincter.

Rectal loading: *see* Faecal loading.

Recto-anal inhibitory reflex: the normal reflex relaxation of the anus in response to rectal distension.

Slow transit constipation: constipation secondary to slow gut transit times.

Third degree tear: tear of the anal sphincter muscles during childbirth.

Whole gut transit time: time taken for ingested items to pass from the mouth to the anus.

1 | Introduction

Jonathan Potter

Consultant Geriatrician, Kent and Canterbury Hospital; Associate Director, Clinical Effectiveness and Evaluation Unit, Royal College of Physicians, London

Bowel care is a major concern to older people.[1] The fear of constipation and the need for regular bowel movements have haunted generations of older people. Equally, the embarrassment associated with faecal incontinence can be one of the greatest threats to personal dignity and quality of life. Despite the prevalence and nature of the condition, older people are frequently loath to complain and seek help.

The importance of the issue was recognised recently with the Department of Health publication *Good Practice in Continence Services*.[2] The publication rightly gives equal weight to the importance of faecal and urinary incontinence. It also demonstrates the impact of faecal incontinence on the individual. The issue has been further highlighted within the National Service Framework (NSF) for Older People,[3] which emphasises the importance of dignity for older people. There are also great costs in terms of management. Bowel care can put great strain on spouses, relatives and carers; it can be the precipitating factor resulting in moving to institutional care; and it has great costs in terms of medications, containment equipment and care.[2]

Despite the clinical prevalence of bowel problems and the cost implications, there is little sound evidence as to the most effective approaches to management. There are no studies of patient-based outcome measures; instead long established treatments are based on anecdote and personal preferences. Studies in older people have been limited and hard to interpret for many methodological reasons. Numbers entered into studies have been low, study groups have not been clearly defined, interventions have often not been randomised or blinded, and outcomes have not been clear. There are persisting problems with definitions and terminology which need to be resolved if meaningful comparisons between studies are to be achieved. Without sound evidence on which to base practice it is not possible to develop appropriate guidelines for management.

In order to move forward in an objective way to improve the management of bowel care, there is a need to define the research evidence as it exists at present. Having done this, it becomes possible to identify areas where further research is needed and, furthermore, to develop guidance on bowel management as far as possible in the light of current knowledge.

The aims of the project detailed in this publication were:

- to initiate a process for more formal evaluation of the evidence base
- to identify the evidence base as it stands at present
- to stimulate research that will clearly answer some of the many questions relevant to bowel care in older people
- to develop pragmatic guidance of use to individuals and carers within the community, in nursing and residential homes, and in hospital settings.

A workshop was organised to undertake this process. Recognised authorities in the field of bowel care were invited to participate, including clinicians with particular expertise in the field as well as representatives of patient and carer groups. A subgroup was asked to review the research evidence, indicate current expert opinion, identify areas where further research is required and outline guidance for practice in selected aspects of care. Their submissions were disseminated to all participants prior to the meeting and were reviewed at the workshop. Participants were asked to indicate if they felt there were any omissions from the literature review and to contribute any further ideas about further research, informed opinion and practice guidance.

The proceedings of the workshop were written up and strength of evidence and recommendations graded according to recognised methods[4] (Appendix 1). The draft document was reviewed by the contributors and the workshop delegates, and also by people suffering from bowel dysfunction or their carers. In this way, a consensus was sought to ensure, first, that the content reflects current knowledge of the issues and, secondly, that the content is pragmatic and relevant to clinicians and individuals concerned or dealing with bowel care.

It is recognised that the methodology does not meet the rigorous criteria required for the formal development of guidelines. The literature review, although detailed, would ideally have been submitted to systematic review using more than one reviewer for each aspect. More detailed consensus arrangements would have been required using, for example, a Delphi exercise[5] to obtain a broader range of opinions, with a subsequent follow-up workshop to refine the findings.

Recurring themes

The process described above identified several recurring themes:

1 There is a crucial issue with regard to *definitions* and *terminology*. These have been debated at length at international meetings with only partial resolution. There are debates as to whether conditions such as constipation and faecal incontinence should be defined on the basis of pathophysiological function, objective symptomatology or subjective determination by the individual requiring care. Until these issues are resolved it will be difficult to obtain clear and meaningful answers from research.

2 There are major issues with regard to *study methodology*. Little useful information can be gathered from current studies because of their small scale and design. Well constructed studies are required, using appropriate qualitative and quantitative methodologies, to provide clear answers.

3 It is important to encourage individuals to *seek help* with regard to bowel care. Furthermore, carers should be trained to recognise bowel problems and to enable older people to discuss such issues without embarrassment. There should be multidisciplinary teams skilled in the assessment and management of this issue and resources available to meet the required needs.

4 *Change and improvement* can be achieved, but important ingredients must be in place if this is to be successful. Carers must buy into the process, for which they need both information about appropriate interventions and support through the process. As demonstrated in Chapter 10, improvements are possible.

5 There are many *myths and anecdotal beliefs* around the use of laxatives, fibre and other approaches to management. The correct place of these different interventions needs to be clarified.

6 Crucially, it is important – and required by the current NSF – that *older people themselves are involved* in the planning of research and its evaluation, and in the development of services that are relevant to them and meet their perceived needs. This is particularly important with regard to bowel care which impinges so importantly not only on physical function but on individual privacy, dignity and quality of life.

The aims of the publication will have been achieved if, first, it contributes to the development of well constructed research into bowel care in older people and, secondly, the guidance given in it in the meantime provides useful advice to individuals and carers so that bowel care can be improved. As clinicians, if we can get the management of bowel care right, we will be a long way towards meeting the principles for providing care for older people enshrined within the NSF.

References

1 Chester R. Feelings and relationships. *Towards Continence*. London: Counsel and Care, 1998.
2 Department of Health. *Good Practice in Continence Services*. PL/CMO/2000/2. London: DH, 2000.
3 Department of Health. *National Service Framework for Older People*. London: DH, 2001.
4 Oxford Centre for Evidence-Based Medicine. *Levels of Evidence and Grades of Recommendations*. http://minerva.minervation.com/cebm/docs/levels.html
5 Gallagher M, Bradshaw C, Nattress H. Policy priorities in diabetes care: a Delphi study. *Qual Health Care* 1996;**5**:3–8.

2 | Pathophysiology of constipation and faecal incontinence in older people

James Barrett
Consultant Physician in Geriatric Medicine and Rehabilitation,
Clatterbridge Hospital, Wirral, Merseyside

Introduction

Research on constipation and faecal incontinence has been mainly performed on young and middle-aged adults, supplemented by some studies on older people. Interest in the subject has been slow to develop but there now appears to be a desire from a number of groups to develop the knowledge base to guide clinical practice. It remains to be seen how the reluctance of some patients and their medical attendants to address this issue can be overcome.

Physiology of bowel function

An outline of the normal anatomy and physiology of the anus and rectum can be found elsewhere.[1,2]

Maintenance of continence

The maintenance of continence is a highly complex process involving not only the anus and rectum but also colonic function which is influenced by diet, physical activity and general health, and the neurological connections from the anorectal area to and from the brain.

The main anorectal mechanisms that contribute towards the maintenance of continence are as follows:

1 The smooth muscle internal anal sphincter maintains anal resting pressure above rectal pressure and thus prevents faecal leakage.[3]
2 The striated (voluntary) muscle external anal sphincter. This makes little contribution to resting pressure,[4] but the reflex response of the sphincter to sudden rectal distension or increased intra-abdominal pressure on standing or coughing helps maintain continence. Voluntary contraction of the external sphincter may also prevent

leakage when there is an urgent desire to defaecate until either the desire wanes or a toilet is found.

3 The anorectal angle is normally 60–105°. Continence may be lost when this angle exceeds 110°.

Other mechanisms which play a role in the maintenance of continence include:

- anal sensation[5]
- the slit shape of the anal canal
- anal cushions – vascular projections which aid closure of the anal canal.[6] Interruption of this mechanism in the treatment of haemorrhoids may lead to incontinence.

Defaecation

Faecal material is presented to the rectum for defaecation by a series of mass movements – often termed the 'gastrocolic response' – the main stimuli for which are physical activity and the ingestion of food.

Faeces in the rectum increase the anorectal angle and cause relaxation of the anal sphincters (the recto-anal inhibitory reflex). This reflex requires an intact myenteric plexus for co-ordinated colonic and rectal motility.

The normal frequency of defaecation varies between three times a day and three times a week and does not appear to change with age.[7] Laxative use is, however, increased in older people, many of whom dread becoming constipated.

Pathophysiology: constipation

Terminology

Constipation is a term used to indicate either the infrequent passage of stool (two or fewer stools passed per week) or excessive straining on attempted defaecation. It may be the presenting symptom of colonic disease.[2]

Read *et al*[8] found that 42% of admissions to acute medical wards for older people were faecally loaded with hard faeces. The presence of constipation in older immobile patients in hospital continuing care beds is related to their mobility, activities of daily living ability, mental status, hearing and speech problems.[9] In one study less than half of older patients who complained of constipation were truly constipated.[10] Straining at stool was the only symptom found to be associated with radiological evidence of colonic faecal loading. The presence of some faeces in the rectum is not necessarily abnormal.

The term 'faecal impaction' is used by many physicians to describe faecal loading of the rectum and/or colon with hard stool. This occurs in patients with a history of chronic constipation but many older patients develop faecal loading with soft stool.[11] Impaction with rock hard stools tends to occur less frequently in disabled older people, accounting for only 10% of the patients in one sample of faecally loaded older patients in rehabilitation and continuing care wards, while 45% had soft or liquid stools and the remainder firm stools.[12] It is therefore more appropriate to use the term 'faecal loading' or 'faecal retention' as the rectum and/or colon may be loaded with a large amount of stool of any consistency. This frequently occurs in older people as a result of an immobilising illness (eg stroke) in the absence of a history of chronic constipation or any other obvious cause.

The presentation of constipation may be atypical as many patients may continue to have a bowel action every day or present with incontinence of urine, faeces or both. Some patients have high faecal loading (ie colonic in the absence of rectal loading). Detection of this may require an abdominal radiograph,[13] but this is generally unnecessary and should not be used routinely.

Pathophysiology

Colonic propulsion

Immobility is an important contributory factor towards the development of both constipation[10,14] and faecal incontinence in older people[12,15] – 30% of immobile older people complain of constipation.[14] The mechanism is likely to be a reduction in colonic mass movements, although no specific studies have been performed to confirm this. A significant reduction in these movements[16] and also in postprandial increase in rectosigmoid motility[17] has been found, while reduced food intake may also reduce colonic propulsive motility.

Whole gut transit time can be measured by serial radiographs following the ingestion of 20 radio-opaque markers. People with a normal transit time pass 80% of the markers within five days.[18] These results are consistent with those from other methods,[19] but they apply only to a Euro-American culture. Shorter transit times have been reported in Africans, suggested by Burkitt et al[20] to be due to their higher dietary fibre intake. Neither colonic transit time[21] nor whole gut transit time appears to change with age, but markedly prolonged transit times have been demonstrated in constipated patients in long-stay geriatric wards, with the markers still *in situ* 14 days after ingestion in 30%.[22] While these patients and many younger constipated patients have slow transit constipation, others have normal transit constipation.

In a study of 28 chronically constipated patients, all of whom had taken laxatives for many years, Preston and Lennard-Jones[23] demonstrated differences between slow transit and normal transit patients. In simulated defaecation studies, slow transit patients were unable to expel a water-filled balloon from the rectum. Their colonic motility traces were normal, although they tended to be rather flat. In contrast, patients with normal transit constipation were able to expel a rectal balloon and were found to have increased colonic activity, which it was suggested might contribute towards the production of small hard stools and the pain they experienced.

A myenteric plexus abnormality has been proposed as a possible cause of slow transit constipation. Evidence of myenteric plexus degeneration has been found in colectomy specimens excised from patients with intractable chronic constipation.[24,25] Preston and Lennard-Jones[26] assessed the myenteric plexus in patients with slow transit constipation by recording the colonic motility response to the direct colonic installation of the stimulant laxative bisacodyl which acts on the myenteric plexus. This produced progressive peristaltic waves in 11 patients but no response in the other seven, and was thought to indicate a myenteric plexus abnormality.

Patients with slow transit constipation therefore appear to be a heterogeneous population. Myenteric plexus degeneration may be the primary cause of their constipation[26] or occur secondary to prolonged laxative use,[24,27] after section of the pelvic nerves[28] and in patients with spinal cord injuries.[29] It may contribute towards constipation in the elderly and/or disabled. A localised defect has now been demonstrated in the enteric nervous system in patients with Parkinson's disease[30,31] in whom gut dysfunction, especially constipation, is common.

The main sites at which gut transit appears to be delayed in older constipated patients are the pelvic colon and rectum.[22] Although mechanical obstruction by impacted faecal masses in the rectum may be the cause of this delay, other mechanisms may operate. A possible generalised enteric nervous system abnormality or abnormal modulation of this system by the central nervous system is suggested by delayed colonic and small bowel transit[32–34] and ileal motility[35] in younger constipated patients.

Defaecatory difficulty

The main purpose of propulsive colonic motility is to present faeces to the rectum for defaecation. Defaecatory abnormalities have been demonstrated in young women with severe slow transit constipation. Many are unable to expel simulated stools from the rectum.[23,36,37] They also experience difficulty expelling barium or saline[38] and may have obstructed defaecation.[39,40]

Normally during defaecation the internal and external anal sphincter and puborectalis muscles relax to allow the passage of stool. Many young constipated people exhibit a paradoxical increase in EMG activity in these muscles during attempted defaecation which obstructs defaecation.[17,23,37,38,41,42]

It has also been suggested that failure of the internal sphincter to relax, as in Hirschsprung's disease,[43] could cause defaecatory difficulty. However, a normal recto-anal inhibitory reflex in response to rectal distension has been demonstrated in both old impacted patients[44] and young chronically constipated patients.[34,37]

Other mechanical causes of obstructed defaecation have been revealed by defaecatory proctography studies of young patients with intractable constipation.[17,45] Roe et al[17] found that 46% of these patients had a rectal intussusception, 12% an anterior rectal wall prolapse, 10% a rectocoele alone and 7% had accentuation of the puborectalis impression. Failure of the anorectal angle to open on defaecatory straining has also been demonstrated in these patients.[17,37,39,46] Although in older impacted patients the angle is obtuse at rest, it appears to increase on straining.[44]

The character of the stool may also cause defaecatory difficulty as even normal individuals find it more difficult to expel small hard stools.[47] Simulated defaecation studies performed on healthy older subjects have revealed that they are able voluntarily to expel a simulated soft stool (50 ml balloon)[8] but require longer to achieve this than younger subjects.[48]

In a study of older patients, all of whom were impacted with hard stool and had been constipated for at least five years, Read et al[8] found that nearly all of them were able to expel a simulated soft stool but experienced difficulty expelling a simulated hard stool (small solid sphere). Only 32% successfully expelled the simulated hard stool compared with 63% of the control group, although this difference did not reach significance. The degree of defaecatory difficulty demonstrated in this study is less than might be expected as many older patients experience it even with soft stools (J A Barrett; personal observations). This appears to be most severe among confused patients who were not included in Read's study group.

Intrarectal pressure normally increases during defaecation with a reduction in anal pressure, producing a pressure gradient which facilitates expulsion of faeces. The increase in intrarectal pressure may be produced by rectal smooth muscle contraction, contraction of the abdominal muscles and diaphragm or by a combination of both.

There appears to be a reduction in rectal motility in old age. Read et al[8] could elicit regular rectal contractions in only 10% of normal older people compared with 71% of a group of young healthy subjects. Only 14% of older impacted patients and 36% of their younger constipated patients exhibited these contractions. These authors suggested that rectal compliance was increased in the older impacted patients, possibly due to a megarectum, but Varma et al[49] were unable to confirm this.

In patients with deficient rectal motility a voluntary increase in intra-abdominal pressure would be expected to produce an increase in intrarectal pressure for defaecation to proceed. This ability is retained in young constipated patients.[36] In some older patients, weakness of the abdominal musculature due either to age-related changes in the muscles (probably secondary to denervation) or to disuse (particularly in immobile patients) could limit this ability, although this has not been studied.

Rectal sensation

Loss of awareness of the call to stool may also contribute towards the development of constipation. Impaired rectal sensation of distension has been demonstrated in patients with chronic constipation,[37] only 38% of whom perceive the desire to defaecate during rectal distension up to 100 ml,[50] and also in older impacted patients.[8,49] Reduced rectal mucosal electrosensitivity has also been demonstrated in constipated patients.[51]

EVIDENCE-BASED SUMMARY ————————————————————

(Strength of evidence [1]–[5]; see Appendix 1)

- Constipation is classically defined as [5]:
  – infrequent passage of stool (two or fewer stools passed per week)
  – passage of hard stool
  – excessive straining on attempted defaecation
  – feeling of incomplete emptying after defaecation.
- Many older people develop faecal loading without having these classic features of constipation [2].
- Constipation may be the presenting symptom of colonic disease [2].
- Whole gut transit time does not change with normal ageing [2].
- Pathophysiological causes of constipation include [2]:
  – abnormalities in colonic propulsion (slow transit time)
  – defaectory difficulty (normal transit time)
  – abnormalities of rectal sensation.

Pathophysiology: faecal incontinence

A number of pathophysiological changes in anorectal function may account for the increased risk of faecal incontinence in older people.

Impaired cognitive function

Impaired consciousness

The most basic requirement for control of bowel evacuation is for a person to be awake. Loss of this will inevitably lead to faecal leakage as voluntary control is not possible. The best example of this type of 'incontinence' occurs in the early stages after a stroke when the level of consciousness is the most important factor determining whether continence is maintained (K J Fullerton: personal communication, from[52]).

Dementia

Many patients with advanced dementia are incontinent of faeces. This may be due to confusion and loss of awareness of the 'call to stool', but other explanations have been sought. Rectal motility is normally under inhibitory cerebral control. This control is absent in many patients with dementia who exhibit uninhibited rectal contractions[53] similar to the uninhibited detrusor contractions that may cause urinary incontinence. These contractions are sufficient to expel a simulated soft stool but not a simulated firm stool.[53] Faecal incontinence occurs when rectal pressure exceeds anal pressure,[3] but the pressure differential may need to be greater for a firm stool to pass.

Behavioural problems

Many patients with severe behavioural problems defaecate in inappropriate places (eg in full view of others in the residents' lounge). This is presumably due to severe frontal lobe damage or degeneration and proves difficult to manage. It may also be associated with faecal smearing and/or coprophagia.

Functional disability

Old age and immobility were found to be associated with an increased risk of faecal incontinence in a multiple regression analysis of the results of the main study of elderly faecally incontinent subjects.[1] This has been reproduced in epidemiological studies of nursing home residents in whom poor mobility is a strong risk factor for faecal incontinence after adjustment for other variables.[54–57] Old age possibly increases the risk of functional disability (because of the age-related changes in bowel and anorectal function described in this chapter) but disability is also an important factor.

There are several reasons why poor mobility may be responsible for an increased chance of faecal incontinence:

▪ It is associated with an increased risk of constipation, as described above.

▪ People who have had a normal bowel habit throughout life can experience severe constipation for the first time when they suffer a disabling illness (eg stroke).

▪ Immobile patients often depend upon others to assist them to a toilet and adjust their clothing in the toilet. They may therefore be slow or reluctant to respond to the call to stool which renders them liable to incontinence – particularly when given a laxative, especially a potent preparation.

Loose stool

Profuse loose stool increases the risk of faecal incontinence in normally continent older adults by overwhelming the continence mechanism. In a prospective nursing home study 44% of cases of faecal incontinence had diarrhoea as a primary cause.[56] In a study of acutely unwell older hospital patients, faecal incontinence was more frequent in patients with loose/liquid stool than in those with hard/soft stools.[58] Multivariate analysis confirmed the strong association of faecal incontinence with unformed/loose or liquid consistency of stool, severe illness and old age.

Anorectal incontinence

Most patients presenting to coloproctology surgical clinics with anorectal incontinence are young or middle-aged women (F:M sex ratio 8:1). The main abnormality is weakness of the anal sphincter and pelvic floor muscles.[59–62] Many patients also have perineal descent,[62,63] but the presence of incontinence is not related to the degree of descent.[40]

Anal endosonography is an ultrasound technique which directly images the anal sphincters and surrounding tissues and is the best method for identifying sphincter defects.[64] On endosonography, the internal sphincter is normally seen as an intact ring. Any break is abnormal and may be due to surgical division[65] or trauma (eg anal dilatation);[66,67] it is usually associated with reduced anal resting pressure.[68,69]

Histological[70,71] and EMG studies[59,72-75] have demonstrated denervation atrophy of the external anal sphincter and puborectalis muscles in these patients. There is also evidence of pudendal neuropathy[59,61,73] and a neuropathy affecting the innervation of puborectalis muscles.[66] Two recent studies of surgical clinic patients suggest that pudendal neuropathy is found more often in patients aged over 50 years than in younger patients, but neither study had a control group.[76,77]

Causes of pudendal neuropathy include stretch injury caused during childbirth or by chronic straining at stool.[78,79] The prevalence of pudendal neuropathy is higher in multigravidae as their pudendal nerve terminal motor latency (PNTML) is more markedly prolonged after vaginal delivery than in primigravidae.[80] Forceps delivery[62] and high infant birthweight[81] increase the risk of pudendal nerve damage. Snooks et al[81] found that two months after delivery this had recovered in 60% of cases, but persistent external sphincter weakness was found in the others when reviewed five years later.[82]

Third-degree obstetric tears are clinically recognised in 1–2% of deliveries, but a prospective study found that 35% of primiparous women had sphincter defects after vaginal delivery when assessed pre- and post-partum with anal endosonography.[83] In 10% of them the sphincter defect was associated with incontinence which was related to the sphincter damage rather than with prolonged PNTML. The risks of sphincter damage are highest when forceps are used. In the Keele randomised controlled trial[84] the risk appeared to be lower with the ventouse vacuum extractor[85] (odds ratio 0.6, 95% confidence interval 0.38–0.97) than with forceps. A follow-up study at five years of just under half the patients randomised in that study found that loss of bowel control was experienced 'sometimes' or 'frequently' by 20%, but there was no difference between the women delivered by the two methods.[86]

The damaged sphincter(s) may start to cause symptoms only in middle age when other factors (eg menopause) are present. Sphincter defects can be found in nearly 90% of patients with anorectal incontinence who have a significant obstetric history.[87,88] Repair of these defects can help to restore continence to these middle-aged women.[89,90]

External anal sphincter weakness with weak anal squeeze

The strength of contraction of the external anal sphincter muscles decreases with age.[48,60,91-93] This appears to be due to denervation[74,94,95] and also occurs in many other muscles in old age.[96] Distal pudendal neuropathy does not appear to account for the age-related weakness.[97] Laurberg and Swash,[92] and Jameson et al[98] have suggested that pudendal nerve latency is related to age, but their data do not support this conclusion. The denervation is more likely to be the result of a central conduction delay, possibly due to age-related loss of either anterior horn cells from the spinal cord or motor nerve fibres from the proximal innervation of the external sphincter.

Reflex contraction of the external sphincter in response to rectal distension is also absent in many older individuals[97] and is deficient in many patients with spinal cord disease.[99,100] Loss of this protective mechanism may contribute towards the increased incidence of faecal incontinence in older people. It does not, however, appear to be related to the degree of external sphincter weakness,[97] although the age-related external sphincter weakness may render older patients liable to the development of faecal incontinence. Even continent older people have external sphincter pressures[97] similar to those recorded in younger, faecally incontinent patients.[61]

Internal sphincter weakness with low anal resting tone

Age does not appear to affect the internal anal sphincter,[91,92,97,99] although some studies purport to demonstrate an age-related reduction in anal resting pressure (internal sphincter pressure).[48,60,93,98] The internal anal sphincter has been shown to increase in thickness with age due to connective tissue replacement of smooth muscle.[67,100] Electron microscopy has demonstrated a less compacted arrangement of the muscle fibres in the elderly, with increased collagen between smooth muscle and stretching of elastic tissue strands.[101]

Significant reduction in anal resting pressure is found in both young[59–61] and elderly faecally incontinent patients[76,97] and is one of the main factors leading to faecal incontinence in frail elderly patients.[12] Normal anal resting pressures have been found in elderly faecally loaded patients[8,44,97] in whom the recto-anal inhibitory reflex can still be elicited.[102]

Anal sensory impairment

Anal sensation is impaired in younger incontinent patients.[5,103,104] It may also be impaired in old age,[97,105] with a greater degree of sensory loss among elderly incontinent patients. Loss of anal sensation, however, does not necessarily result in faecal incontinence. Read and Read[106] demonstrated that continence can be maintained when the anal canal is anaesthetised with lignocaine gel, suggesting that continence may be lost only when a number of coexistent abnormalities are present.

Colorectal faecal loading

Faecal loading is the most common cause of faecal incontinence in older people. Faecal soiling in faecally loaded patients is more common when soft stool is present. Many of these incontinent patients leak before they experience a call to stool,[53] probably due to anal sphincter relaxation before the onset of rectal sensation[107] and to the absence of the reflex external sphincter contraction in response to rectal distension.[108]

Although rectal sensation is impaired in older impacted patients,[8,43,49] it does not appear to account for their incontinence.[5,12,109] Anal sphincter weakness and loss of the anorectal angle appear to be contributory factors.[43] Faecal incontinence may also be produced by the treatment of faecal loading in immobile patients.

Comorbidity-related faecal incontinence

This topic is discussed in Chapter 3.

EVIDENCE-BASED SUMMARY ————————————————————

(*Strength of evidence* [1]–[5]; see Appendix 1)

The pathophysiological causes of faecal incontinence are [2]:

- impaired cognitive function
- impaired physical function
- loose stools
- colorectal faecal loading
- anorectal incontinence
- comorbidity.

WHAT WE DON'T KNOW

- Questions remain unanswered about the anorectal physiology of bowel problems in old age. These include:
  - Why is anal resting tone lower in older people with faecal incontinence?
  - What happens to the anal sphincters as ageing occurs? It seems that the external sphincter becomes weaker but the internal sphincter does not; and is childbirth as important a factor?
  - Why is faecal loading with soft faeces so prevalent in frail old people?
  - Why is lactose malabsorption more common in people aged 60–79 years than in those aged 40–59 years?

- What is the effect of ageing on the physiology of defaecation, and what factors may cause defaecatory difficulty in later life?

■ More work is needed to refine the definition and terminology associated with faecal incontinence:

- Is incontinence of flatus a real problem or just a minor social embarrassment?
- Does slight faecal staining of the underwear constitute faecal incontinence or a variation of normal?
- Does a problem exist only when there is involuntary passage of a significant amount of faeces?

■ Future studies in older people will need to define carefully the setting in which they are undertaken. There are likely to be differences between the reasons for faecal incontinence in acutely ill older people and those in the community or in long-term care. Patients with primary psychiatric illness probably comprise another separate group.

■ Valid and reliable measurement instruments are required for bowel symptoms and their severity. Those currently in use do not always adequately describe the problem: for example, the faecally loaded and incontinent older person usually has a large amount of soft faeces in the rectum that leaks many times per day but does not fit the classical definition of constipation on the grounds of the frequency of passing stool, the need to strain or the passage of hard stool.

■ A comprehensive longitudinal cohort study is required to delineate the natural history of bowel dysfunction in the community.

■ What is the pathophysiological relationship in older people between continence and such factors as diet, physical activity, general health and the neurological connections between the anorectal area and the brain?

■ Are there any factors in young and middle age that increase the risk of faecal incontinence in old age? If so, could they be avoided/prevented? Possible contenders include:

- diet
- medications, especially laxatives
- surgical procedures
- obstetric and gynaecological factors
- gastrointestinal disease
- disability
- mental state
- psychiatric state

- IQ (faecal incontinence is common in people with learning disabilities)
- sexuality
- level of physical activity.

▪ What is the usefulness of sophisticated tests of anorectal function in the management of the older patient in comparison with basic clinical history and physical examination?

▪ What leads sufferers of faecal incontinence to seek help or prevents them from seeking help? It appears that many do not seek help although they will discuss a problem with 'diarrhoea'.

▪ Is loss of bowel control a poor prognostic sign for survival in some conditions in old age (eg stroke)?

References

1 Barrett JA. *Faecal Incontinence in the Older Adult.* London: Edward Arnold, 1993.
2 Barrett JA, Chew D. Disorders of the lower gastrointestinal tract. *Rev Clin Gerontol* 1991;**1**:119–34.
3 Read NW, Haynes WG, Bartolo DC, Hall J *et al.* Use of anorectal manometry during rectal infusion of saline to investigate sphincter function in incontinent patients. *Gastroenterology* 1983;**85**:105–13.
4 Frenckner B, Euler CV. Influence of pudendal block on the function of the anal sphincters. *Gut* 1975;**16**:482–9.
5 Rogers J, Henry MM, Misiewicz JJ. Combined sensory and motor deficit in primary neuropathic faecal incontinence. *Gut* 1988;**29**:5–9.
6 Gibbons CP, Trowbridge EA, Bannister JJ, Read NW. Role of anal cushions in maintaining continence. *Lancet* 1986;**i**:886–8.
7 Connell AM, Hilton C, Irvine G, Lennard-Jones JE, Misiewicz JJ. Variation of bowel habits in two population samples. *BMJ* 1965;**2**:1095–9.
8 Read NW, Abouzekry L, Read MG, Howell P *et al.* Anorectal function in elderly patients with fecal impaction. *Gastroenterology* 1985;**89**:959–66.
9 Resende TL. *Constipation, faecal incontinence and the effects of exercise and abdominal massage on colonic activity in old age.* MSc thesis, University of Manchester, 1989.
10 Donald IP, Smith RG, Cruikshank JG, Elton RA, Stoddart ME. A study of constipation in the elderly living at home. *Gerontology* 1985;**31**:112–8.
11 Barrett JA. Effect of wheat bran on stool size. *BMJ* 1988;**296**:1127–8.
12 Barrett JA. *A study of the pathophysiology of faecal incontinence among geriatric patients.* MD thesis, University of Liverpool, 1988.
13 Smith RG, Lewis S. The relationship between digital rectal examination and abdominal radiographs in elderly patients. *Age Ageing* 1990;**19**:142–3.
14 Whitehead WE, Drinkwater D, Cheskin LJ, Heller BR, Schuster MM. Constipation in the elderly living at home. Definition, prevalence, and relationship to lifestyle and health status. *J Am Geriatr Soc* 1989;**37**:423–9.
15 Barrett JA, Faragher EB, Kiff ES, Ferguson G, Brocklehurst JC. Why are geriatric patients incontinent of faeces? *Clin Sci* 1988;**75**(Suppl 19):10P.
16 Bassotti G, Gaburri M, Imbimbo B, Peli MA, Morelli A. Colonic mass movements in health and in constipation. *Gastroenterology* 1987;**92**:1310.

17   Roe AM, Bartolo DC, Mortensen NJ. Diagnosis and surgical management of intractable constipation. *Br J Surg* 1986;**73**:854–61.

18   Hinton JM, Lennard-Jones JE, Young AC. A new method for studying gut transit times using radioopaque markers. *Gut* 1969;**10**:842–7.

19   Cummings JH, Jenkins DJ, Wiggins HS. Measurement of the mean transit time of dietary residue through the human gut. *Gut* 1976;**17**:210–8.

20   Burkitt DP, Walker AR, Painter NS. Effect of dietary fibre on stools and the transit-times, and its role in the causation of disease. *Lancet* 1972;**ii**:1408–12.

21   Meier R, Beglinger C, Dederding JP, Meyer-Wyss B *et al.* Influence of age, gender, hormonal status and smoking habits on colonic transit time. *Neurogastroenterol Motil* 1995;**7**:235–8.

22   Brocklehurst JC, Kirkland JL, Martin J, Ashford J. Constipation in long-stay elderly patients: its treatment and prevention by lactulose, poloxalkol-dihydroxyanthroquinolone and phosphate enemas. *Gerontology* 1983;**29**:181–4.

23   Preston DM, Lennard-Jones JE. Anismus in chronic constipation. *Dig Dis Sci* 1985;**30**:413–8.

24   Preston DM, Butler MG, Smith B, Lennard-Jones JE. Neuropathology of slow transit constipation. *Gut* 1983;**24**:A997.

25   Krishnamurthy S, Schuffler MD, Rohrmann CA, Pope CE 2nd. Severe idiopathic constipation is associated with a distinctive abnormality of the colonic myenteric plexus. *Gastroenterology* 1985;**88**:26–34.

26   Preston DM, Lennard-Jones JE. Pelvic motility and response to intraluminal bisacodyl in slow-transit constipation. *Dig Dis Sci* 1985;**30**:289–94.

27   Smith B. Effect of irritant purgatives on the myenteric plexus in man and the mouse. *Gut* 1968;**9**:139–43.

28   Devroede G, Lamarche J. Functional importance of extrinsic parasympathetic innervation to the distal colon and rectum in man. *Gastroenterology* 1974;**66**:273–80.

29   Devroede G, Arhan P, Duguay C, Tetreault L *et al.* Traumatic constipation. *Gastroenterology* 1979;**77**:1258–67.

30   Singaram C, Ashraf W, Gaumnitz EA, Torbey C *et al.* Dopaminergic defect of enteric nervous system in Parkinson's disease patients with chronic constipation. *Lancet* 1995;**346**:861–4.

31   Bassotti G, Maggio D, Battaglia E, Giulietti O *et al.* Manometric investigation of anorectal function in early and late stage Parkinson's disease. *J Neurol Neurosurg Psychiatry* 2000;**68**:768–70.

32   Youle MS, Read NW. Effect of painless rectal distension on gastrointestinal transit of solid meal. *Dig Dis Sci* 1984;**29**:902–6.

33   Kellow JE, Gill RC, Wingate DL. Modulation of human upper gastrointestinal motility by rectal distension. *Gut* 1987;**28**:864–8.

34   Bannister JJ, Timms JM, Barfield LJ, Donnelly TC, Read NW. Physiological studies in young women with chronic constipation. *Int J Colorectal Dis* 1986;**1**:175–82.

35   Panagamuwa B, Kumar D, Ortiz J, Keighley MR. Motor abnormalities in the terminal ileum of patients with chronic idiopathic constipation. *Br J Surg* 1994;**81**:1685–8.

36   Barnes PR, Lennard-Jones JE. Balloon expulsion from the rectum in constipation of different types. *Gut* 1985;**26**:1049–52.

37   Read NW, Timms JM, Barfield LJ, Donnelly TC, Bannister JJ. Impairment of defecation in young women with severe constipation. *Gastroenterology* 1986;**90**:53–60.

38 Turnbull GK, Lennard-Jones JE, Bartram CI. Failure of rectal expulsion as a cause of constipation: why fibre and laxatives sometimes fail. *Lancet* 1986;**i**: 767–9.

39 Preston DM, Lennard-Jones JE, Thomas BM. The balloon proctogram. *Br J Surg* 1984;**71**:29–32.

40 Bartolo DC, Read NW, Jarratt JA, Read MG, *et al.* Differences in anal sphincter function and clinical presentation in patients with pelvic floor descent. *Gastroenterology* 1983;**85**:68–75.

41 Womack NR, Williams NS, Holmfield JH, Morrison JF, Simpkins KC. New method for the dynamic assessment of anorectal function in constipation. *Br J Surg* 1985;**72**:994–8.

42 Kuijpers HC, Bleijenberg G, de Morree HD. The spastic pelvic floor syndrome. Large bowel outlet obstruction caused by pelvic floor dysfunction: a radiological study. *Int J Colorectal Dis* 1986;**1**:44–8.

43 Lawson JO, Nixon HH. Anal canal pressures in the diagnosis of Hirschsprung's disease. *J Paediatr Surg* 1967;**2**:544–52.

44 Read NW, Abouzekry L. Why do patients with faecal impaction have faecal incontinence? *Gut* 1986;**27**:283–7.

45 Bartolo DC, Roe AM, Virjee J, Mortensen NJ. Evacuation proctography in obstructed defaecation and rectal intussusception. *Br J Surg* 1985;**72**(Suppl): S111–6.

46 Womack NR, Morrison JFB, Williams NS. The role of pelvic floor denervation in the aetiology of idiopathic faecal incontinence. *Br J Surg* 1986;**73**:404–7.

47 Bannister JJ, Davison P, Timms JM, Gibbons C, Read NW. Effect of stool size and consistency on defecation. *Gut* 1987;**28**:1246–50.

48 Bannister JJ, Abouzekry L, Read NW. Effect of aging on anorectal function. *Gut* 1987;**28**:353–7.

49 Varma JS, Bradnock J, Smith RG, Smith AN. Constipation in the elderly. A physiologic study. *Dis Colon Rectum* 1988;**31**:111–5.

50 Kerrigan DD, Lucas MG, Sun WM, Donelly TC, Read NW. Idiopathic constipation associated with impaired urethrovesical and sacral reflex function. *Br J Surg* 1989;**76**:748–51.

51 Kamm MA, Lennard-Jones JE. Rectal mucosal electrosensory testing – evidence of a rectal sensory neuropathy in idiopathic constipation. *Dis Colon Rectum* 1990;**33**:419–23.

52 Fullerton KJ, Mackenzie G, Stout RW. Prognostic indices in stroke. *Q J Med* 1988;**66**:147–62.

53 Barrett JA, Brocklehurst JC, Kiff ES, Ferguson G, Faragher EB. Rectal motility studies in faecally incontinent geriatric patients. *Age Ageing* 1990;**19**:311–7.

54 Chassagne P, Landrin I, Neveu C, Czernichow P *et al.* Fecal incontinence in the institutionalized elderly: incidence, risk factors, and prognosis. *Am J Med* 1999;**106**:185–90.

55 Nelson R, Norton N, Cautley E, Furner S. Community-based prevalence of anal incontinence. *JAMA* 1995;**274**:559–61.

56 Johanson JF, Irizarry F, Doughty A. Risk factors for fecal incontinence in a nursing home population. *J Clin Gastroenterol* 1997;**24**:156–60.

57 Chiang L, Ouslander J, Schnelle J, Reuben DB. Dually incontinent nursing home residents: clinical characteristics and treatment differences. *J Am Geriatr Soc* 2000;**48**:673–6.

58 Bliss DZ, Johnson S, Savik K, Clabots CR, Gerding DN. Fecal incontinence in hospitalized patients who are acutely ill. *Nurs Res* 2000;**49**:101–8.

59 Snooks SJ, Henry MM, Swash M. Anorectal incontinence and rectal prolapse:

differential assessment of the innervation to puborectalis and external anal sphincter muscles. *Gut* 1985;**26**:470–6.

60 Read NW, Harford WV, Schmulen AC, Read MG *et al.* A clinical study of patients with fecal incontinence and diarrhea. *Gastroenterology* 1979;**76**: 747–56.

61 Kiff ES, Swash M. Slowed conduction in the pudendal nerves in idiopathic (neurogenic) faecal incontinence. *Br J Surg* 1984;**71**:614–6.

62 Snooks SJ, Henry MM, Swash M. Faecal incontinence due to external anal sphincter division in childbirth is associated with damage to the innervation of the pelvic floor musculature: a double pathology. *Br J Obstet Gynaecol* 1985;**92**:824–8.

63 Read NW, Bartolo DC, Read MG. Differences in anal function in patients with incontinence to solids and in patients with incontinence to liquids. *Br J Surg* 1984;**71**:39–42.

64 Bartram CI, Sultan AH. Anal endosonography in faecal incontinence. Review. *Gut* 1995;**37**:4–6.

65 Sultan AH, Kamm MA, Nicholls RJ, Bartram CI. Prospective study of the extent of internal anal sphincter division during lateral sphincterotomy. *Dis Colon Rectum* 1994;**37**:1031–3.

66 Speakman CT, Burnett SJ, Kamm MA, Bartram CI. Sphincter injury after anal dilatation demonstrated by anal endosonography. *Br J Surg* 1991;**78**:1429–30.

67 Nielsen MB, Hauge C, Rasmussen OO, Sorensen M *et al.* Anal sphincter size measured by endosongraphy in healthy volunteers. Effect of age, sex, and parity. *Acta Radiol* 1992;**33**:453–6.

68 Felt-Bersma RJ, Cuesta MA, Koorevaar M, Strijers RL *et al.* Anal endo-sonography: relationship with anal manometry and neurophysiologic tests. *Dis Colon Rectum* 1992;**35**:944–9.

69 Falk PM, Blatchford GJ, Cali RL, Christensen MA, Thorson AG. Transanal ultrasound and manometry in the evaluation of faecal incontinence. *Dis Colon Rectum* 1994;**37**:468–72.

70 Parks AG, Swash M, Urich H. Sphincter denervation in anorectal incon-tinence and rectal prolapse. *Gut* 1977;**18**:656–65.

71 Beersiek F, Parks AG, Swash M. Pathogenesis of ano-rectal incontinence. A histometric study of the anal sphincter musculature. *J Neurol Sci* 1979;**42**: 111–27.

72 Neill ME, Parks AG, Swash M. Physiological studies of the anal sphincter musculature in faecal incontinence and rectal prolapse. *Br J Surg* 1981;**68**: 531–6.

73 Kiff ES, Swash M. Normal proximal and delayed distal conduction in the pudendal nerves of patients with idiopathic (neurogenic) faecal incontinence. *J Neurol Neurosurg Psychiatry* 1984;**47**:820–3.

74 Bartolo DCC, Jarratt JA, Read NW. The use of conventional electro-myography to assess external sphincter neuropathy in man. *J Neurol Neurosurg Psychiatry* 1983;**46**:1115–8.

75 Bartolo DC, Jarratt JA, Read MG, Donnelly TC, Read NW. The role of partial denervation of the puborectalis in idiopathic faecal incontinence. *Br J Surg* 1983;**70**:664–7.

76 Rasmussen OO, Christiansen J, Tetzschner T, Sorensen M. Pudendal nerve function in idiopathic fecal incontinence. *Dis Colon Rectum* 2000;**43**:633–6; discussion 636–7.

77 Vaccaro CA, Cheong DM, Wexner SD, Nogueras JJ *et al.* Pudendal neuro-pathy in evacuatory disorders. *Dis Colon Rectum* 1995;**38**:166–71.

78 Kiff ES, Barnes PR, Swash M. Evidence of pudendal neuropathy in patients with perineal descent and chronic straining at stool. *Gut* 1984;**25**:1279–82.

79 Snooks SJ, Barnes PR, Swash M, Henry MM. Damage to the innervation of the pelvic floor musculature in chronic constipation. *Gastroenterology* 1985;**89**: 977–81.

80 Snooks SJ, Swash M, Henry MM, Setchell M. Risk factors in childbirth causing damage to the pelvic floor innervation. *Br J Surg* 1985;**72**(Suppl): S15–7.

81 Snooks SJ, Setchell M, Swash M, Henry MM. Injury to innervation of pelvic floor sphincter musculature in childbirth. *Lancet* 1984;**ii**:546–50.

82 Snooks SJ, Swash M, Mathers SE, Henry MM. Effect of vaginal delivery on the pelvic floor: a 5-year follow-up. *Br J Surg* 1990;**77**:1358–60.

83 Sultan AH, Kamm MA, Hudson CN, Thomas JM, Bartram CI. Anal-sphincter disruption during vaginal delivery. *N Engl J Med* 1993;**329**:1905–11.

84 Sultan AH, Kamm MA, Bartram CI, Hudson CN. Anal sphincter trauma during instrumental delivery. *Int J Gynaecol Obstet* 1993;**43**:263–70.

85 Johanson RB, Rice C, Doyle M, Arthur J *et al.* A randomised prospective study comparing the new vacuum extractor policy with forceps delivery. *Br J Obstet Gynaecol* 1993;**100**:524–30.

86 Johanson RB, Heycock E, Carter J, Sultan AH *et al.* Maternal and child health after assisted vaginal delivery: five-year follow up of a randomised controlled study comparing forceps and ventouse. *Br J Obstet Gynaecol* 1999;**106**:544–9.

87 Burnett SJD, Spence-Jones C, Speakman CT, Kamm MA *et al.* Unsuspected sphincter damage following childbirth revealed by anal endosonography. *Br J Radiol* 1991;**64**:225–7.

88 Deen KI, Kumar D, Williams JG, Olliff J, Keighley MR. The prevalence of anal sphincter defects in faecal incontinence: a prospective endosonic study. *Gut* 1993;**34**:685–8.

89 Engel AF, Kamm MA, Sultan AH, Bartram CI, Nicholls RJ. Anterior anal sphincter repair in patients with obstetric trauma. *Br J Surg* 1994;**81**:1231–4.

90 Nielsen MB, Dammegaard L, Pedersen JF. Endosonographic assessment of the anal sphincter after surgical reconstruction. *Dis Colon Rectum* 1994;**37**:434–8.

91 Matheson DM, Keighley MRB. Manometric evaluation of rectal prolapse and faecal incontinence. *Gut* 1981;**22**:126–9.

92 Laurberg S, Swash M. Effects of aging on the anorectal sphincters and their innervation. *Dis Colon Rectum* 1989;**32**:737–42.

93 McHugh SM, Diamant NE. Effect of age, gender, and parity on anal canal pressures. Contribution of impaired anal sphincter function to fecal incontinence. *Dig Dis Sci* 1987;**32**:726–36.

94 Percy JP, Neill ME, Kandiah TK, Swash M. A neurogenic factor in faecal incontinence in the elderly. *Age Ageing* 1982;**11**:175–9.

95 Neill ME, Swash M. Increased motor unit fibre density in the external anal sphincter muscle in ano-rectal incontinence: a single fibre EMG study. *J Neurol Neurosurg Psychiatry* 1980;**43**:343–7.

96 Grimby G, Saltin B. The ageing muscle. Review. *Clin Physiol* 1983;**3**:209–18.

97 Barrett JA, Brocklehurst JC, Kiff ES, Ferguson G, Faragher EB. Anal function in geriatric patients with faecal incontinence. *Gut* 1989;**30**:1244–51.

98 Jameson JS, Chia YW, Kamm MA, Speakman CT *et al.* Effect of age, sex and parity on anorectal function. *Br J Surg* 1994;**81**:1689–92.

99 Loening-Baucke V, Anuras S. Anorectal manometry in healthy elderly subjects. *J Am Geriatr Soc* 1984;**32**:636–9.

100 Burnett SJ, Bartram CI. Endosonographic variations in the normal internal anal sphincter. *Int J Colorectal Dis* 1991;**6**:2–4.

101 Swash M, Gray A, Lubowski DZ, Nicholls RJ. Ultrastructural changes in internal anal sphincter in neurogenic faecal incontinence. *Gut* 1988;**29**:1692–8.

102 Tobin GW. Incontinence in the elderly. *Practitioner* 1987;**231**:843–4, 847.

103 Roe AM, Bartolo DC, Mortensen NJ. New method for assessment of anal sensation in various anorectal disorders. *Br J Surg* 1986;**73**:310–2.

104 Miller R, Bartolo DC, Cervero F, Mortensen NJ. Anorectal temperature sensation: a comparison of normal and incontinent patients. *Br J Surg* 1987;**74**:511–5.

105 Ryhammer AM, Laurberg S, Bek KM. Age and anorectal sensibility in normal women. *Scand J Gastroenterol* 1997;**32**:278–84.

106 Read NW, Read MG. Role of anal sensation in preserving continence. *Gut* 1982;**23**:345–7.

107 Buser WD, Miner PB Jr. Delayed rectal sensation with fecal incontinence. Successful treatment using anorectal manometry. *Gastroenterology* 1986;**91**:1186–91.

108 Wald A, Tunuguntla AK. Anorectal sensorimotor dysfunction in fecal incontinence and diabetes mellitus. Modification with biofeedback therapy. *N Engl J Med* 1984;**310**:1282–7.

109 Ferguson GH, Redford J, Barrett JA, Kiff ES. The appreciation of rectal distension in fecal incontinence. *Dis Colon Rectum* 1989;**32**:964–7.

3 | Epidemiology and risk factors for bowel problems in older people

Danielle Harari

Senior Lecturer in Elderly Medicine, St Thomas' Hospital Elderly Care Unit,
Guy's, King's and St Thomas' Hospital School of Medicine, London

Epidemiology of constipation in older people

Introduction

Constipation is a frequent health concern for older people and their healthcare providers. The number of physician visits for constipation increases markedly among people over 65 years[1,2] as does regular laxative use.[3] The self-reported symptom of constipation has been associated with anxiety, depression and poor health perception, while clinical constipation in frail older individuals may lead to serious complications such as faecal impaction and overflow, sigmoid volvulus and urinary retention.

Quality of data

The applied definitions of constipation in older people in the epidemiological literature have been inconsistent. Studies tend to define constipation:

- subjectively by self-report
- according to specific bowel-related symptoms or
- by daily laxative usage.

Few epidemiological studies use an objective assessment-based definition.[4] Only one of the risk factor studies reviewed was prospective;[5] the remainder are retrospective studies with reasonable sample sizes and adjusted odds ratio analysis (unless noted otherwise). Other data regarding causes are derived from publications in which constipation was assessed as a potential associated factor with a primary condition (eg Parkinson's disease, drug adverse effect).

Definition of constipation

The feeling of being constipated will often mean different things to different individuals. Until five years ago, the non-specific and subjective

23

definition of 'self-reported' constipation was used in epidemiological studies of older people. Based on international consensus and recently updated, constipation is now defined according to self-report of more specific bowel-related symptoms ('Rome II criteria').[6] The following definition for *functional constipation* is useful both in practice and in clinical research:

> Two or more of the following symptoms on more than 25% of occasions in the prior three months: two or less bowel movements per week, hard stool, straining, feeling of incomplete evacuation (prevalence rate of 24% among community-dwellers aged over 65).[7]

An important subtype of constipation is *rectal outlet delay* which affects 21% of community-dwellers aged 65 and over. It is defined as:

> Feeling of anal blockage during evacuation and prolonged defaecation (>10 min) and/or need for manual evacuation.[7]

While less subjective than self-reported constipation ('Do you feel constipated?'), these two definitions are nevertheless patient-oriented and symptom-based. Objectively, however, the clinical definition of constipation relies on evidence of excessive stool retention in the rectum and/or colon. Such objective assessment is particularly important in frail older people who may:

- be unable to report bowel-related symptoms due to communication or cognitive difficulties
- have regular bowel movements despite having rectal or colonic stool impaction
- have impaired rectal sensation and rectal dyschezia and so be unaware of symptoms associated with a large faecal bolus in the rectum[8]
- have non-specific symptoms (such as delirium, leucocytosis, anorexia, functional decline) in association with severe faecal impaction.

Prevalence of constipation and constipation-related symptoms

Self-reported constipation

The generally held belief that constipation is an inevitable consequence of ageing stems partly from questionnaire-based studies which found a marked increase of self-reported constipation with age. One community-based study (n = 3,166) asked people aged 65 and over 'Do you have recurrent constipation?' and found a prevalence of 26% in women and 16% in men, with a prevalence of 34% and 26%, respectively, in the over 84 age group.[9] Age was a strong independent risk factor for self-reported constipation. Other community studies support the relationship of age with self-reported constipation, and show prevalence rates of up to 34% in women and 30% in men over 65.[3,4,10,11] The preponderance of women over men reporting constipation tends to reduce beyond the age of 80 years.[3,10,12]

Infrequent bowel movements

In contrast, the weekly frequency of bowel movements does not alter with ageing alone,[3,13] with only 1–7% of both young and older community-dwelling individuals reporting frequency below the normal range (two or less bowel movements a week).[3,10,13,14] This consistent bowel pattern across age groups persists even after statistical adjustment for the greater amount of laxatives used by older people.[3] Community-based studies of older people show that less than 10% of those complaining of constipation report two or fewer weekly bowel movements and over half move their bowels daily.[10,15] However, physical frailty in older persons increases the risk of self-report of infrequent bowel movements (two or less bowel movements a week):[4,16]

- 17% of nursing home residents[12]
- 14% of geriatric day hospital patients[4]
- 33% of long-term care residents.[12]

Difficult evacuation

The implication is that bowel-related symptoms other than infrequent bowel movements also drive self-reporting of constipation in older persons. These symptoms are primarily straining and passage of hard stools.[4,7,10,15] In a US community study, 65% of older people reporting constipation had persistent straining and 39% passage of hard bowel movements.[15] Constipated older people tend to suffer chiefly from difficulties with rectal evacuation, as shown by a prevalence rate of 21% for rectal outlet delay among community-dwelling people aged 65 and over.[7] Another study found that 30% of nursing home residents reported persistent straining.[12]

Constipation symptoms in the long-term care setting

In a Finnish study,[17] Kinnunen found a prevalence of constipation (defined as self-reported difficult evacuation or infrequent bowel movements) of 57% in women and 64% in men living in residential homes, and 79% and 81%, respectively, in the nursing home setting. The high prevalence of constipation in the latter is all the more striking in that 50–74% of long-term care residents use one or more daily laxatives.[12,17–19] Advancing age has been shown to be an independent risk factor for heavy laxative use[19] and for symptom-based constipation[17] among older nursing home patients. Evidence mainly from case-series suggests that complications of constipation such as faecal impaction,[11] overflow,[8,12] constipation-related hospital admission,[8] sigmoid volvulus and bladder outlet obstruction[20] are more likely to affect frailer older people.

EVIDENCE-BASED SUMMARY

(*Strength of evidence* [1]–[5]; see Appendix 1)

- The prevalence of both self-reported constipation and symptomatic constipation is high in frail older people [2].

- Self-reported constipation increases in prevalence with advancing age [2].

- Women predominate over men in prevalence rates of self-reported constipation and related symptoms among older people, though this gender difference is less marked beyond the age of 80 [2].

- Bowel movement frequency does not alter with ageing alone, even after adjustment for increased laxative use by older people [2].

- Constipated older people tend to suffer primarily from difficulties with rectal evacuation and symptoms of straining and hard stool [2].

- Nursing home residents have a higher prevalence than community-dwelling individuals of all constipation-related symptoms, including infrequent bowel movements, straining and hard stool [2].

- Advancing age increases the risk for heavy laxative use and symptom-based constipation among nursing home patients [3].

- The prevalence of constipation in nursing homes is high despite heavy laxative usage [2] implying that:
  - laxative prescribing may be ineffective
  - non-pharmacological approaches to treatment are underutilised in this setting
  - frail older people are at greater risk of faecal impaction and other complications of constipation [3].

Risk factors for constipation in older people

Robson *et al* looked prospectively at baseline characteristics predictive of new-onset constipation in older nursing home patients (n = 1,291), using the US Minimum Data Set instrument.[5] Constipation was defined as having two or fewer bowel movements per week or straining on more than 25% of occasions. They found that 7% developed constipation over a three-month period. Independent predictors were white race, poor consumption of fluids, pneumonia, Parkinson's disease, decreased mobility, more than five medications, dementia, hypothyroidism, allergies, arthritis and hypertension. The authors postulated that the last three were associated primarily because of the constipating effect of drugs used to treat these conditions. Other research data regarding risk factors for constipation are presented below.

Polypharmacy

The risk of constipation in older patients[5,9,10,17] is increased by polypharmacy, particularly in nursing homes where each individual takes an average of six prescribed medications per day.[12] Overall, constipation as a drug side effect is likely to be substantially under-reported in older people.

Drug side effects

Certain classes of drugs are particularly implicated in promoting constipation.

Anticholinergics Drugs with strong anticholinergic properties reduce gut smooth muscle contractility via an antimuscarinic effect at acetylcholine receptor sites; in some cases, long-term use may induce chronic colonic dysmotility. In two cross-sectional studies of nursing home residents, anticholinergic antidepressants were independently associated with daily laxative use (following adjustment for age, gender, function and cognition).[19,21] Anticholinergic neuroleptics and antihistamines were also independently associated in one of the studies.[19] Non-anticholinergic sedatives were not found to be constipating.

Opiate analgesia Older people are highly susceptible to the constipating effects of opiate analgesia. Individuals over 60 have higher plasma concentrations of beta-endorphin with increased binding to endogenous opiate receptors in the gut.[22] This may exacerbate the opiate effect of relaxing colonic tone, reducing motility and inhibiting the gastrocolic reflex in older people receiving opiates for pain. Parenthetically, it has been reported that naloxone given to nursing home residents with constipation can result in an increase in stool output and a reduction in constipation symptoms.[22]

Iron supplements All types of iron supplements (sulphate, fumarate and gluconate) have the same propensity to cause constipation in adults, though slow-release wax-matrix preparations may have a lesser impact on the large bowel.[23]

Calcium-channel antagonists   Severe constipation has been reported in older patients taking calcium-channel antagonists. Nifedipine and verapamil are more potent inhibitors of gut motility than diltiazem and newer agents.[24]

Non-steroidal anti-inflammatory drugs   The risk of constipation in older people is increased with the use of non-steroidal anti-inflammatory drugs (NSAIDs),[11] probably through prostaglandin inhibition. In a large case-controlled primary care study, constipation and straining were more common in NSAID users, and constipation was a more common reason for stopping medication than dyspepsia.[25] These studies did not, however, adjust for the possible confounder of arthritis impacting mobility.

Other risk factors for constipation

Immobility   Immobility is a primary risk factor for constipation.[4,17,21] In the long-term care setting, Kinnunen[17] found that 89% of bed- or chair-bound patients were constipated compared with 44% of those walking more than 0.5 km per day and that immobility was strongly associated with an increased risk of constipation. Donald *et al*[4] found that poor mobility among geriatric outpatients was covariantly associated with symptom-based constipation.

These studies particularly examined ambulatory immobility as a risk factor, but it is likely that problems of sensory and dexterity impairment may also contribute. Exercise in bed and the use of abdominal massage have been shown to reduce laxative and enema use in chair-fast geriatric long-stay patients although transit time was unaffected.[26]

Institutionalisation   Institutionalisation itself is an independent risk factor for symptom-based constipation.[17]

Parkinson's disease   In older patients, Parkinson's disease may cause severe constipation symptoms.[5,21] Patients suffer from dual pathologies of:

▪ primary degeneration of dopaminergic neurons in the enteric nervous system, resulting in prolonged transit throughout the entire gut,[27] and

▪ pelvic dyssynergia, resulting in rectal outlet delay and prolonged straining even early in the course of the disease.[27,28]

Diabetes mellitus   A survey of outpatients in a diabetic clinic found that 60% complained of constipation.[29] Those with autonomic neuropathy are more likely to be affected due to markedly slowed transit throughout the colon.[30]

Low fluid intake Low fluid intake in older adults has been related to symptomatic constipation.[5,31] Withholding fluids over a one-week period in young male volunteers significantly reduced stool output.[32] Elderly people are at greater risk of dehydration due to impaired thirst sensation and less effective hormonal responses to hypertonicity, while those in nursing homes and hospitals may also have functional reasons for being unable to drink.

Dietary fibre The intake of dietary fibre is often low in older people[10] but no clear association has been made with clinical constipation in this population. In younger, healthy constipated adults, low dietary fibre has been associated (through meta-analysis) with increased stool weight and decreased transit time.[33] One community study in older subjects found that higher fibre intake correlated with lower laxative use amongst older women,[34] but in another study higher intake of bran was associated with no reduction in constipation symptoms and greater faecal loading in the colon on abdominal radiography.[4] Four small uncontrolled nursing home studies have suggested that daily bran fibre increases bowel movement frequency, reduces laxative intake and the need for nursing intervention in frail older persons.[35–38] However, concomitant increased fluid intake may have contributed significantly to these positive results.

Dementia The presence of dementia predisposes individuals to rectal dyschezia,[8,39] possibly partly through ignoring the urge to defaecate. A study in which young men deliberately suppressed defaecation resulted in prolonged transit through the rectosigmoid, with a marked reduction in frequency of bowel movements.[40] Epidemiological studies have found no significant association between cognitive impairment and symptomatic constipation,[10,17] though it has been associated with nurse-documented constipation in the nursing home.[5]

Psychological problems Depression, psychological distress and anxiety are all associated with increased self-reporting of constipation in older persons.[10,41] The symptom of constipation is sometimes a somatic manifestation of psychiatric illness. A careful assessment is required to differentiate subjective complaints and clinical constipation in depressed or anxious patients.

Spinal cord disease or injury Constipation is a significant clinical problem in most people with spinal cord disease or injury.[42,43] Age and duration of injury interact to promote complications of chronic constipation such as acquired megacolon which affects over half of patients with spinal cord injury.[42]

Metabolic imbalance   Metabolic imbalances of hypothyroidism, uraemia, hypokalaemia and hypercalcaemia should not be overlooked as remediable causes of clinical constipation.

Colorectal cancer   Colon cancer is associated with both constipation and use of laxatives, though this risk association is likely to be confounded by the influence of underlying habits.[44] The prevalence of colorectal cancer increases with age, so the index of suspicion should be higher in older adults. Abdominal pain, rectal bleeding, recent change in bowel habit and any systemic features (eg weight loss, anaemia) should prompt further investigations for underlying neoplasm.[45]

EVIDENCE-BASED SUMMARY ─────────────────────────

(*Strength of evidence* [1]–[5]; see Appendix 1)

▮ There are numerous potentially modifiable risk factors for constipation in frail older people [2].
▮ Risk factors for symptomatic constipation in older people are:
  – polypharmacy [2]
  – anticholinergic drugs [2]
  – opiate analgesia [2]
  – iron supplements [3]
  – calcium-channel antagonists [2]
  – NSAIDs [2]
  – immobility [2]
  – institutionalisation [3]
  – Parkinson's disease [2]
  – diabetes mellitus [2]
  – low fluid intake [2]
  – low dietary fibre intake [3]
  – dementia [2]
  – depression and other psychological problems [3]
  – spinal cord disease or injury [2]
  – hypothyroidism [2]
  – uraemia, hypokalaemia, hypercalcaemia [3].

▮ Certain symptoms associated with constipation (abdominal pain, rectal bleeding, recent change in bowel habit, weight loss, anaemia) should prompt further investigations for underlying neoplasm [2].

WHAT WE DON'T KNOW

▮ Why is the prevalence of constipation in nursing homes so high despite heavy laxative usage? Is it, for example:
  – ineffective laxative prescribing?
  – suboptimal assessment of patients?
  – underuse of non-pharmacological treatment approaches?
▮ How can standardised 'constipation protocols' for case-finding and risk assessment be implemented across community and institutional healthcare settings where frail older patients are cared for?
▮ How feasible is the widespread use of a nursing instrument for clinical assessment (where nurses collect data that trigger management pathways) of bowel problems in frail older people living in UK nursing homes? Such approaches are widely used in nursing homes in the USA (eg Minimum Data Set).[46]
▮ Randomised controlled trials are needed to assess the impact of non-pharmacological interventions targeting constipation risk factors on bowel and health-related outcomes in frail older people.
▮ Common evidence-based policies, procedures, guidelines and targets are required to promote integrated bowel care for frail older people. This emphasises the need for further research into this area – and the need for awareness among grant-issuing bodies of the importance of funding this type of research.

Epidemiology of faecal incontinence in older people

Introduction

Few medical symptoms are as distressing and socially isolating for older people as faecal incontinence, a condition which places them at greater risk of morbidity, mortality, dependency, hospital admissions and institutionalisation. Many older individuals in the community with faecal incontinence will not volunteer the problem to their general practitioner (GP) and, regrettably, doctors and nurses do not routinely enquire about the symptom. This 'hidden problem' therefore leads to social isolation and a downward spiral of psychological distress, dependency and poor health. Even when older people are noted by healthcare professionals to have faecal incontinence, the condition is often managed passively, especially in the long-term care setting where it is most prevalent. The importance of identifying risk factors in order to treat underlying causes of faecal incontinence, rather than just applying conservative management, is strongly emphasised in the Department of Health (DH) report, *Good Practice in Continence Services.*[47]

Epidemiological studies

Quality of data

There is a lack of standardisation in defining faecal incontinence among epidemiological studies in older adults; this creates opportunities for misclassifications of the condition and hampers cross-study comparisons. Most community-based studies examine the prevalence of faecal incontinence occurring at least once over the previous year. This may overestimate the prevalence of significant symptoms, but provides the upper limit for faecal incontinence in this population. Long-term care studies mostly measure weekly or monthly occurrence. None of the epidemiological studies in older adults used faecal incontinence scoring systems such as the Wexner score (which includes use of pads, impact on lifestyle, consistency and frequency of faecal incontinence).[48,49] The Wexner score is the most widely used scale in clinical research, but the data are presently insufficient to support its universal use as a standard-ised grading system for faecal incontinence, particularly as it has not been validated for use in older people.

The studies reviewed include one prospective short-term cohort study,[50] while all the others were retrospectively conducted surveys. Risk factor analyses were unadjusted in some studies[18,51] and retrospectively conducted in all but one.[52] The epidemiology of faecal incontinence in older adults varies according to the general health of the study population, so the studies were presented according to the setting in which the work was conducted (community, hospital or nursing home).

Results

Community-dwelling persons   A US survey of 2,400 randomly selected individuals aged 50 years and above found a faecal incontinence prevalence (one or more episode in the past year) of 11% in men and 15% in women.[53] Prevalence increased significantly with age in men (from 8% to 18% between the sixth and ninth decade) but not in women. Half those reporting faecal incontinence also reported urinary incontinence. A similar US survey reported a prevalence of 2% (the definition for faecal incontinence included uncontrolled passage of gas) for a population aged 18 and upwards. Old age was independently associated with faecal incontinence in a subgroup analysis, but not as strongly as physical limitations and poor general health.[54]

There was a 9% prevalence of faecal incontinence among 527 Irish primary care patients aged 75 years and over, one in six of whom was experiencing daily incontinence.[55]

A community-based study from Japan showed a 2% prevalence of daily faecal incontinence in people over 65 years (n = 1,405), with 9% of men and 7% of women reporting 'some degree' of faecal incontinence.[56] In the over 85 age group, 29% of women and 25% of men (or their carers) reported faecal incontinence, the great majority also having urinary incontinence. Independent risk factors for faecal incontinence were:

I age older than 75 years

I poor general health (measured as activities of daily living dependency)

I stroke

I dementia

I no participation in social activities, and

I a feeling that there is not much to live for.

The authors followed up this cohort after 42 months and found that severe faecal incontinence (at least once weekly) was associated with increased mortality, independent of age, gender and poor general health.[57]

Hospital inpatients In a British survey of 627 hospitalised patients aged 65 and over, in which faecal incontinence was defined as at least one episode weekly, there was a 14% prevalence.[51] An Australian survey of 247 consecutively acutely hospitalised patients of all ages found that 22% self-reported faecal incontinence.[58]

Long-term care residents Chassagne *et al*[52] documented a baseline prevalence of faecal incontinence of 54% among 2,602 nursing home residents in France. Over a 10-month period there was a 20% incidence of new-onset faecal incontinence in those who were continent at baseline; faecal incontinence was transient (<5 days) in 62% of these, and long-standing in 38%. Faecal incontinence was equally prevalent in women and men. Of the patients who developed long-standing incontinence, 26% died within 10 months compared with 7% of those who remained continent. Independent correlates of new-onset faecal incontinence were age over 70 years, urinary incontinence, neurological disease, poor mobility and impaired cognitive function.

A recent survey by Brocklehurst *et al*[18] of 498 nursing home residents in England living in 21 long-term care facilities showed that faecal incontinence occurred at least once weekly in 29% and less frequently in a further 23% (a total of 52% incontinent at some time). Faecal incontinence was significantly more common in men.

Another British survey of at least once weekly incontinence in institutionalised adults aged 65 and over found a 13% prevalence rate in residential homes and up to 37% in nursing home residents.[51] In these UK studies there was a wide variation between individual nursing homes in the prevalence of faecal incontinence (17–95%).[18,51,59] The case-mix within these nursing homes is likely to be comparable, so the variations may be more reflective of different standards of care than of different patient characteristics. The strongest univariate associations with faecal incontinence in these long-term care studies were physical dependency and impaired mobility, particularly where help was needed to transfer from bed to chair.[18,51]

Faecal incontinence prevalence rates of 17–46% have been documented in US and Canadian nursing homes.[12,50] Johanson *et al*[50] documented independent risk factors for faecal incontinence in nursing home residents as frequent diarrhoea, watery stool, dementia, restricted mobility, and male gender.

Faecal incontinence in older adults: the 'hidden' problem

In a British primary care study of patients aged 75 years and over, only half those reporting faecal incontinence (or their carers) had discussed the problem with a healthcare professional, and only one out of eight patients with daily incontinence. The GPs involved in this study reported full knowledge of incontinence status in only 33% of patients with a continence problem.[55] In an Australian survey of acutely hospitalised patients of all ages, only one in six of those reporting faecal incontinence had the symptom documented by ward nursing staff.[57]

A US nursing home study showed that nursing staff were aware of faecal incontinence in only 53% of residents self-reporting the condition.[12] The kappa value for concordance between resident and nurse reporting of faecal incontinence was only 0.34 (95% confidence interval 0.24–0.43).

In Tobin and Brocklehurst's study of nursing home residents, only 4% of patients with long-standing faecal incontinence had been referred to their GP for further assessment of this problem.[59]

EVIDENCE-BASED SUMMARY

(*Strength of evidence* [1]–[5]; see Appendix 1)

■ The prevalence of faecal incontinence increases with age alone, particularly in the eighth decade and beyond [2].

■ The prevalence of faecal incontinence is higher in the acute hospital and nursing home setting than in the community [2]. The impact of the condition is therefore greatest in frailer older people.

■ Unlike younger populations, the prevalence of faecal incontinence in frail older people is equal to or greater in men than in women [2]. This predominance is most striking among nursing home residents. The pathophysiology underlying these findings in men is yet to be explored.

■ The prevalence of faecal incontinence varies dramatically among institutions in British nursing home studies [2]. Further research is needed to examine underlying reasons for these variations (eg standards of care, patient case-mix, reporting).

■ Faecal incontinence is often combined with urinary incontinence in frail older people [2].

■ In addition to age, primary risk factors for faecal incontinence in older people are impaired mobility, dementia, neurological disease and loose stool [2].

■ Physicians and nurses in primary care, acute hospital and long-term care healthcare settings have a low awareness of faecal incontinence in older people [2].

■ Within nursing homes, there is a low rate of referral by nursing staff of residents to their primary care physicians for further assessment of faecal incontinence [2]. This may reflect a tendency toward conservative nursing management (eg use of pads alone, without further evaluation).

Causes of faecal incontinence in older people

The causes of faecal incontinence in older people, unlike in younger adults, are often multifactorial. The aim of this section is to categorise faecal incontinence in the frail older adult by primary cause in a clinically meaningful way, emphasising the identification of potentially reversible factors. A classification of faecal incontinence is shown in Box 1 and discussed below.

Box 1. Classification of faecal incontinence (from presentations by J Barrett, D Harari and C Norton)

A Faecal incontinence related to colorectal faecal loading:
Immobility
Medication side effects:
   iron supplements
   calcium supplements
   calcium channel antagonists
   non-steroidal anti-inflammatory drugs
   opiates
   drugs with anticholinergic effects, eg:
      – tricyclic antidepressants
      – antipsychotics
      – anti-Parkinsonian medication
      – oxybutynin
Parkinson's disease
Low dietary intake
Low fluid intake
Dementia

B Faecal incontinence related to functional disability:
Patient related:
   poor mobility
   poor dexterity
   poor vision
Carer related:
   availability
   attitude
Related to suitability of toilet facility/toileting ability

C Faecal incontinence due to loss of cognitive awareness:
Impaired consciousness
Dementia
Behavioural

D Faecal incontinence related to comorbidity:
Stroke
Diabetes mellitus
Spinal cord dysfunction:
   multiple sclerosis
   spinal cord injury
Parkinson's disease
Autonomic dysfunction
Systemic sclerosis

continued

Box 1 continued

E Anorectal incontinence:
Anal sphincter degeneration
Anal sphincter and/or pudendal nerve disruption:
    childbirth
    anal surgery
    anal stretch
    traumatic injury
    hysterectomy/previous surgery
    chronic straining at stool
    unwanted anal penetration
    anal sexual use
Idiopathic

F Faecal incontinence related to loose stools:
Carcinoma of the rectum or colon
Laxative related
Fibre related
Antibiotic-related diarrhoea
Medication side effects
Infectious diarrhoea:
    rotavirus infections
    Clostridium difficile
    salmonella
    campylobacter
Colitis:
    inflammatory bowel disease
    ischaemic
    radiotherapy induced
Lactose intolerance
Malabsorption
Bacterial overgrowth in small bowel

Overflow incontinence secondary to constipation and stool impaction

Constipation is the most important cause of faecal incontinence in frail older people; it is treatable, preventable and frequently overlooked. Read *et al*[8] reported that faecal impaction was a primary reason for acute hospitalisation in 27% of geriatric patients admitted over the course of a year. The prevalence of faecal impaction with overflow incontinence is high in nursing home patients. Although there are no studies examining overflow in the community for comparative purposes, it is likely that institutionalisation places older individuals at greater risk of the condition. Tobin and Brocklehurst[59] identified overflow (continuous faecal soiling and faecal impaction on rectal examination) as the underlying problem in

52% of frail nursing home residents with long-standing faecal incontinence. A therapeutic intervention consisting of enemas until no further response followed by lactulose achieved complete resolution of incontinence in 94% of those in whom full treatment compliance could be obtained.[59] Another study of frail nursing home patients found that a regimen of daily lactulose and suppositories plus weekly enemas was effective in resolving overflow faecal incontinence only when long-lasting and complete rectal emptying was achieved.[60]

There are almost no published data on causes of impaction and overflow, but there are data on risk factors for constipation in older adults. These are detailed in the section above on Risk factors for constipation.

Functional incontinence

Functional incontinence occurs in individuals who are unable to access the toilet in time due to impairments in mobility, dexterity or vision. These patients may even have normal lower gut function. Epidemiological studies of nursing home residents (see above) have repeatedly shown that poor mobility is a strong risk factor for faecal incontinence after adjustment for other variables.[50,52,54,57]

Dementia-related incontinence

Patients with advanced dementia may have a neurologically disinhibited rectum, with a tendency to void formed stool once or twice daily following mass peristaltic movements. Tobin and Brocklehurst[59] documented dementia as the primary cause of faecal incontinence in 46% of nursing home residents, and the condition has been identified as an independent risk factor in epidemiological studies.[50,52,57] These individuals are commonly also incontinent of urine.[57]

Comorbidity-related incontinence

The following diseases may cause faecal incontinence and are more common in older people.

Stroke

Immediately following a stroke 40% of individuals are incontinent, and 10% remain so six months after the acute event.[61] There are few data examining the pathophysiological basis for faecal incontinence following stroke. In a multivariate adjusted analysis faecal incontinence in three-month stroke survivors was shown to be more strongly associated with potentially modifiable factors of anticholinergic medication use and functional difficulties in getting to the toilet, rather than with stroke severity or location.[62]

Diabetes mellitus

Faecal incontinence may occur in people with diabetic neuropathy affecting the gut through the dual mechanisms of:

▪ bacterial overgrowth resulting from severe prolongation of gut transit causing the characteristic nocturnal diarrhoea, and

▪ multifactorial anorectal dysfunction.[63]

Case-control studies show that diabetic patients with faecal incontinence have reduced basal and squeeze pressures, spontaneous relaxation of the internal anal sphincter, reduced rectal compliance, and abnormal rectal sensation.[63,64]

Sacral cord dysfunction

The neuropathophysiology of rectal dyschezia[8] is compatible with diminished parasympathetic outflow from the sacral cord. Rectal dyschezia is clinically associated with recurrent rectal impaction and continuous faecal soiling.[8] It is characterised by:

▪ impaired rectal sensation (needing a larger volume before feeling the presence of a rectal balloon and the urge to void)

▪ lower rectal pressures during rectal distension

▪ impaired anal and perianal sensation.

Common conditions in older persons that could impair sacral cord function are ischaemia and spinal stenosis.

Anorectal incontinence

Studies of older people with faecal incontinence suggest that age-related internal anal sphincter dysfunction is an important contributing factor[65,66] as it lowers the threshold for balloon (stimulated stool) expulsion.[65] Childbearing is linked to faecal incontinence in later life via structural damage to the external anal sphincter and pelvic musculature.[67] Pudendal neuropathy is an age-related phenomenon in women with faecal incontinence, but has an unclear role as a predisposing factor for incontinence.[66,68] Rectal prolapse is also a cause of faecal incontinence which occurs more commonly in older adults.[69] Prior anal surgery has not been identified as a risk factor in surveys of faecal incontinence in community-dwellers,[54] but certain procedures such as sphincterotomy for fissure *in ano* and fistulotomy have an 8% and 18–52% risk of faecal incontinence, respectively, in patients of all ages.[70,71]

Loose stool

Loose stool increases the risk of incontinence in normally continent older adults by overwhelming a functional but age-compromised sphincter mechanism. Frail older individuals are particularly susceptible to bowel leakage in the context of loose stools.[52,59] In a prospective nursing home study 44% of cases of faecal incontinence were related primarily to acute diarrhoea.[52]

Potentially reversible causes

Loose stools should be considered a possible indicator of serious underlying disease such as neoplasm or colitis, and all patients with this symptom should be screened clinically for systemic illness. Where a change in bowel habit is identified, colonoscopy should be considered to rule out colorectal cancer.[72] There are, however, several potentially reversible causes of loose stool in frail older adults.

Excessive use of laxatives   One-third of community-dwelling people aged 65 and over regularly take laxatives, far exceeding the prevalence of constipation in this population, thus implying overuse.[3] In the nursing home setting, laxative use (in particular 'Codanthramer') has been linked to faecal incontinence.[18]

Drug side effects   Proton-pump inhibitors, selective serotonin re-uptake inhibitors and magnesium-containing antacids are examples of drugs associated with loose stool.

Lactose intolerance   This is an age-related phenomenon. Goulding *et al*[73] found a 15% lactose malabsorption rate in healthy women aged 40–59 years compared with 50% in those aged 60–79.

Antibiotic-related diarrhoea   Among hospitalised patients, age, female gender and nursing home residency significantly increase the risk for *Clostridium difficile*-associated diarrhoea related to antibiotic use.[74] The diarrhoea also takes longer to resolve following treatment of *C. difficile* in frailer older patients.

EVIDENCE-BASED SUMMARY ─────────────────────────────

(*Strength of evidence* [1]–[5]; see Appendix 1)

■ Overflow incontinence secondary to stool impaction is a primary cause of faecal incontinence in nursing home residents [3].

- There are multiple potentially modifiable causes of constipation in older people [2]; they are likely to be risk factors also for overflow incontinence [4].
- Frail older people may be incontinent because they are unable to use the toilet for functional reasons [2].
- Dementia-related faecal incontinence is an important cause of bowel leakage in frail older people [2].
- Faecal incontinence is a common complication following stroke [2], but factors other than stroke status itself are contributory causes for incontinence in stroke survivors [3].
- Loose stool predisposes older people to soiling [2] and has numerous potentially reversible causes [3]. Loose stool may, however, be indicative of underlying colonic disease such as colorectal cancer or colitis and patients with this symptom should be carefully evaluated [2].

WHAT WE DON'T KNOW

- Consensus agreement on a standardised definition of faecal incontinence in older people would be useful in both clinical and research arenas. A proposed definition is that used in the DH report, *Good Practice in Continence Services:*[47]

  involuntary or inappropriate passing of faeces that has an impact on social functioning or hygiene.

- Why is there variability of faecal incontinence rates among British nursing homes, even taking into consideration case-mix issues? Different institutional standards of care may affect the occurrence of the condition. National audit of current practice in long-term care is needed to lay the groundwork for standardised care.
- What are the processes for the identification of faecal incontinence in older primary care patients? An audit of current processes of case-finding in primary care (by GPs, practice nurses and continence nurse specialists) would be useful.
- What is the feasibility of 'intermediate care' centres, offering an opportunity for primary care physicians, continence nurse specialists and geriatricians to provide an integrative approach to the assessment of the faecally incontinent older person, in accordance with the National Service Framework for Older People recommendations?[75]
- Further epidemiological studies are required to document causes of faecal incontinence in frail older people in different healthcare

settings. Such studies should include evaluation of unmet need for patients and carers.

∎ Why is there a high prevalence of faecal incontinence in older men? An exploration of aetiologies other than childbirth in ageing adults is required.

∎ Further work is needed to evaluate potentially preventable causes of loose stools in institutionalised older people.

References

1 Petticrew M, Watt I, Sheldon T. Systematic review of the effectiveness of laxatives in the elderly. Review. *Health Technol Assess* 1997;**1**:i–iv,1–52.

2 Sonnenberg A, Koch TR. Physician visits in the United States for constipation: 1958 to 1986. *Dig Dis Sci* 1989;**34**:606–11.

3 Harari D, Gurwitz JH, Avorn J, Bohn R, Minaker KL. Bowel habits in relation to age and gender. Findings from the National Health Interview Survey and clinical implications. *Arch Intern Med* 1996;**156**:315–20.

4 Donald IP, Smith RG, Cruikshank JG, Elton RA, Stoddart ME. A study of constipation in the elderly living at home. *Gerontology* 1985;**31**:112–8.

5 Robson KM, Kiely DK, Lembo T. Development of constipation in nursing home residents. *Dis Colon Rectum* 2000;**43**:940–3.

6 Thompson WG, Longstreth GF, Drossman DA, Heaton KW *et al.* Functional bowel disorders and functional abdominal pain. Review. *Gut* 1999; **45**(Suppl 2): II43–7.

7 Talley NJ, O'Keefe EA, Zinsmeister AR, Melton LJ 3rd. Prevalence of gastrointestinal symptoms in the elderly: a population-based study. *Gastroenterology* 1992;**102**:895–901.

8 Read NW, Abouzekry L, Read MG, Howell P *et al.* Anorectal function in elderly patients with fecal impaction. *Gastroenterology* 1985;**89**:959–66.

9 Stewart RB, Moore MT, Marks RG, Hale WE. Correlates of constipation in an ambulatory elderly population. *Am J Gastroenterol* 1992;**87**:859–64.

10 Whitehead WE, Drinkwater D, Cheskin LJ, Heller BR, Schuster MM. Constipation in the elderly living at home. Definition, prevalence, and relationship to lifestyle and health status. *J Am Geriatr Soc* 1989;**37**:423–9.

11 Talley NJ, Fleming KC, Evans JM, O'Keefe EA *et al.* Constipation in an elderly community: a study of prevalence and potential risk factors. *Am J Gastroenterol* 1996;**91**:19–25.

12 Harari D, Gurwitz JH, Avorn J, Choodnovskiy I, Minaker KL. Constipation: assessment and management in an institutionalized elderly population. *J Am Geriatr Soc* 1994;**42**:947–52.

13 Everhart JE, Go VL, Johannes RS, Fitzsimmons SC *et al.* A longitudinal survey of self-reported bowel habits in the United States. *Dig Dis Sci* 1989;**34**: 1153–62.

14 Milne JS, Williamson J. Bowel habit in older people. *Gerontol Clin (Basel)* 1972; **14**:56–60.

15 Harari D, Gurwitz JH, Avorn J, Bohn R, Minaker KL. How do older persons define constipation? Implications for therapeutic management. *J Gen Intern Med* 1997;**12**:63–6.

16 Campbell AJ, Busby WJ, Horwath CC. Factors associated with constipation in a community based sample of people aged 70 years and over. *J Epidemiol Community Health* 1993;**47**:23–6.

17 Kinnunen O. Study of constipation in a geriatric hospital, day hospital, old people's home and at home. *Aging (Milano)* 1991;**3**:161–70.
18 Brocklehurst J, Dickinson E, Windsor J. Laxatives and faecal incontinence in long-term care. *Nurs Stand* 1999;**13**:32–6.
19 Monane M, Avorn J, Beers MH, Everitt DE. Anticholinergic drug use and bowel function in nursing home patients. *Arch Intern Med* 1993;**153**:633–8.
20 Knobel B, Rosman P, Gewurtz G. Bilateral hydronephrosis due to fecaloma in an elderly woman. Review. *J Clin Gastroenterol* 2000;**30**:311–3.
21 Harari, D, Gurwitz JH, Choodnovskiy I, Minaker KL. Correlates of regular laxative use by frail elderly persons. *Am J Med* 1995;**99**:513–8.
22 Szurszewski JH, Holt PR, Schuster M. Proceedings of a workshop, entitled 'Neuromuscular function and dysfunction of the gastrointestinal tract in aging'. *Dig Dis Sci* 1989;**34**:1135–46.
23 Brock C, Curry H, Hanna C, Knipfer M, Taylor L. Adverse effects of iron supplementation: a comparative trial of a wax-matrix iron preparation and conventional ferrous sulfate tablets. *Clin Ther* 1985;**7**:568–73.
24 Traube M, McCallum RW. Calcium-channel blockers and the gastrointestinal tract. American College of Gastroenterology's Committee on FDA related matters. Review. *Am J Gastroenterol* 1984;**79**:892–6.
25 Jones RH, Tait CL. Gastrointestinal side-effects of NSAIDs in the community. *Br J Clin Pract* 1995;**49**:67–70.
26 Resende TL, Brocklehurst JC, O'Neill PA. A pilot study on the effect of exercise and abdominal massage on bowel habit in continuing care patients. *Clin Rehabil* 1993;**7**:204–9.
27 Edwards LL, Quigley EM, Pfeiffer RF. Gastrointestinal dysfunction in Parkinson's disease: frequency and pathophysiology. Review. *Neurology* 1992;**42**: 726–32.
28 Bassotti G, Maggio D, Battaglia E, Giulietti O *et al.* Manometric investigation of anorectal function in early and late stage Parkinson's disease. *J Neurol Neurosurg Psychiatry* 2000;**68**:768–70.
29 Feldman M, Schiller LR. Disorders of gastrointestinal motility associated with diabetes mellitus. Review. *Ann Intern Med* 1983;**98**:378–84.
30 Camilleri M. Gastrointestinal problems in diabetes. Review. *Endocrinol Metab Clin North Am* 1996;**25**:361–78.
31 Towers AL, Burgio KL, Locher JL, Merkel IS *et al.* Constipation in the elderly: influence of dietary, psychological, and physiological factors. *J Am Geriatr Soc* 1994;**42**:701–6.
32 Klauser AG, Schindlbeck NE, Muller-Lissner SA. Low fluid intake lowers stool output in healthy male volunteers. *Z Gastroenterol* 1990;**28**:606–9.
33 Muller-Lissner SA. Effect of wheat bran on weight of stool and gastrointestinal transit time: a meta analysis. *BMJ* 1988;**296**:615–7.
34 Johnson CK, Kolasa K, Chenoweth W, Bennink M *et al.* Health, laxation, and food habit influences on fiber intake of older women. *J Am Diet Assoc* 1980;**77**:551–7.
35 Valle-Jones JC. An open study of oat bran meal biscuits ('Lejfibre') in the treatment of constipation in the elderly. *Curr Med Res Opin* 1985;**9**: 716–20.
36 Pringle R, Pennington MJ, Pennington CR, Ritchie RT. A study of the influence of a fibre biscuit on bowel function in the elderly. *Age Ageing* 1984;**13**:175–8.
37 Hull C, Greco RS, Brooks DL. Alleviation of constipation in the elderly by dietary fiber supplementation. *J Am Geriatr Soc* 1980;**28**:410–4.

38 Hope AK, Down EC. Dietary fibre and fluid in the control of constipation in a nursing home population. *Med J Aust* 1986;**144**:306–7.

39 Barrett JA, Brocklehurst JC, Kiff ES, Ferguson G, Faragher EB. Anal function in geriatric patients with faecal incontinence. *Gut* 1989;**30**:1244–51.

40 Klauser AG, Voderholzer WA, Heinrich CA, Schindlbeck NE, Muller-Lissner SA. Behavioral modification of colonic function. Can constipation be learned? *Dig Dis Sci* 1990;**35**:1271–5.

41 Garvey M, Noyes R Jr, Yates W. Frequency of constipation in major depression: relationship to other clinical variables. *Psychosomatics* 1990;**31**: 204–6.

42 Harari D, Minaker KL. Megacolon in patients with chronic spinal cord injury. Review. *Spinal Cord* 2000;**38**:331–9.

43 Hinds JP, Eidelman BH, Wald A. Prevalence of bowel dysfunction in multiple sclerosis. A population survey. *Gastroenterology* 1990;**98**:1538–42.

44 Sonnenberg A, Muller AD. Constipation and cathartics as risk factors of colorectal cancer: a meta-analysis. *Pharmacology* 1993;**47**(Suppl 1):224–33.

45 Majumdar SR, Fletcher RH, Evans AT. How does colorectal cancer present? Symptoms, duration, and clues to location. *Am J Gastroenterol* 1999;**94**: 3039–45.

46 Morris JN, Lipsitz LA, Murphy K, Belleville-Taylor P (eds). *Quality Care in the Nursing Home*. St Louis: Mosby Lifeline, 1997.

47 Department of Health. *Good Practice in Continence Services*. PL/CMO/2000/2. London: NHS Executive, 2000.

48 Jorge JMN, Wexner SD. Etiology and management of fecal incontinence. Review. *Dis Colon Rectum* 1993;**36**:77–97.

49 Vaizey DJ, Carapeti E, Cahill JA, Kamm MA. Prospective comparison of faecal incontinence grading systems. *Gut* 1999;**44**:77–80.

50 Johanson JF, Irizarry F, Doughty A. Risk factors for fecal incontinence in a nursing home population. *J Clin Gastroenterol* 1997;**24**:156–60.

51 Peet SM, Castleden CM, McGrother CW. Prevalence of urinary and faecal incontinence in hospitals and residential and nursing homes for older people. *BMJ* 1995;**311**:1063–4.

52 Chassagne P, Landrin I, Neveu C, Czernichow P *et al*. Fecal incontinence in the institutionalized elderly: incidence, risk factors, and prognosis. *Am J Med* 1999;**106**:185–90.

53 Roberts RO, Jacobsen SJ, Reilly WT, Pemberton JH *et al*. Prevalence of combined fecal and urinary incontinence: a community-based study. *J Am Geriatr Soc* 1999;**47**:837–41.

54 Nelson R, Norton N, Cautley E, Furner S. Community-based prevalence of anal incontinence. *JAMA* 1995;**274**:559–61.

55 Prosser S, Dobbs F. Case-finding incontinence in the over-75s. *Br J Gen Pract* 1997;**47**:498–500.

56 Nakanishi N, Tatara K, Naramura H, Fujiwara H *et al*. Urinary and fecal incontinence in a community-residing older population in Japan. *J Am Geriatr Soc* 1997;**45**:215–9.

57 Nakanishi N, Tatara K, Shinsho F, Murakami S, *et al*. Mortality in relation to urinary and faecal incontinence in elderly people living at home. *Age Ageing* 1999;**28**:301–6.

58 Schultz A, Dickey G, Skoner M. Self-report of incontinence in acute care. Review. *Urol Nurs* 1997;**17**:23–8.

59 Tobin GW, Brocklehurst JC. Faecal incontinence in residential homes for the elderly: prevalence, aetiology and management. *Age Ageing* 1986;**15**:41–6.

60 Chassagne P, Jego A, Gloc P, Capet C *et al*. Does treatment of constipation

improve faecal incontinence in institutionalized elderly patients. *Age Ageing* 2000;**29**:159–64.

61 Nakayama H, Jorgensen HS, Pedersen PM, Raaschou HO, Olsen TS. Prevalence and risk factors of incontinence after stroke. The Copenhagen Stroke Study. *Stroke* 1997;**28**:58–62.

62 Harari D, Coshall C, Rudd SG, Wolfe CDA. New-onset faecal incontinence following stroke: prevalence, natural history, risk factors and impact. *Stroke* 2002 (in press).

63 Wald A, Tunuguntla AK. Anorectal sensorimotor dysfunction in fecal incontinence and diabetes mellitus. Modification with biofeedback therapy. *N Engl J Med* 1984;**310**:1282–7.

64 Sun WM, Katsinelos P, Horowitz M, Read NW. Disturbances in anorectal function in patients with diabetes mellitus and faecal incontinence. *Eur J Gastroenterol Hepatol* 1996;**8**:1007–12.

65 Barrett JA, Brocklehurst JC, Kiff ES, Ferguson G, Faragher EB. Rectal motility studies in faecally incontinent geriatric patients. *Age Ageing* 1990;**19**:311–7.

66 Rasmussen OO, Christiansen J, Tetzschner T, Sorensen M. Pudendal nerve function in idiopathic fecal incontinence. *Dis Colon Rectum* 2000;**43**:633–6; discussion 636–7.

67 Nygaard IE, Rao SS, Dawson JD. Anal incontinence after anal sphincter disruption: a 30 year retrospective study. *Obstet Gynecol* 1997;**89**:896–901.

68 Vaccaro CA, Cheong DM, Wexner SD, Nogueras JJ *et al.* Pudendal neuropathy in evacuatory disorders. *Dis Colon Rectum* 1995;**38**:166–71.

69 Matheson DM, Keighley MR. Manometric evaluation of rectal prolapse and faecal incontinence. *Gut* 1981;**22**:126–9.

70 Pernikoff BJ, Eisenstat TE, Rubin RJ, Oliver GC, Salvati EP. Reappraisal of partial lateral internal sphincterotomy. *Dis Colon Rectum* 1994;**37**:1291–5.

71 Del Pino A, Nelson RL, Pearl RK, Abcarian H. Island flap anoplasty for treatment of transsphincteric fistula-in-ano. *Dis Colon Rectum* 1996;**39**:224–6.

72 Colon cancer screening (USPSTF) recommendations. US Preventive Services Task Force. *J Am Geriatr Soc* 2000;**48**:333–5.

73 Goulding A, Taylor RW, Keil D, Gold E *et al.* Lactose malabsorption and rate of bone loss in older women. *Age Ageing* 1999;**28**:175–80.

74 Al-Eidan FA, McElnay JC, Scott MG, Kearney MP. Clostridium difficile-associated diarrhoea in hospitalised patients. *J Clin Pharm Ther* 2000;**25**:101–9.

75 Department of Health. *National Service Framework for Older People.* London: DH, 2001.

4 | Assessing the individual

Christine Norton
Nurse Consultant (Bowel Control), St Mark's Hospital, North West London Hospitals NHS Trust, Harrow; Honorary Professor of Nursing, King's College, London

James Barrett
Consultant Physician in Geriatric Medicine and Rehabilitation, Clatterbridge Hospital, Wirral, Merseyside

Clinical symptoms

No evidence-based assessment protocols have been published for bowel problems in older people. Informed opinion suggests that taking a history and performing a physical examination are the most important parts of the assessment process. Older people frequently do not report their bowel problems.[1,2] However, when they do, they are shown to be reliable with self-reporting of bowel symptoms[3,4] though clinicians may fail to take an accurate history or perform a rectal examination.[5] Perhaps history taking should be preceded by completion of a symptom questionnaire by the patients.[6]

Bowel problems in these older patients are often multifactorial. An assessment proforma including the most important areas for assessment[7] is shown in Box 1. The following components should be included in the assessment:

- bowel habit (past and present)
- diet, with questions specifically about fibre intake
- awareness of call to stool
- the process of defaecation, including evacuation difficulty
- stool consistency, for which the Bristol stool chart[8] can help to clarify the type of stools passed – no research data are available for older people, but younger patients can reliably evaluate their own stool consistency[9]
- episodes of leakage – younger adults, patients with predominantly external anal sphincter weakness, report urgency prior to leak, while those with internal sphincter dysfunction tend to be unaware of stool leakage[10]

Box 1. Assessment of faecal incontinence and constipation checklist (adapted from Ref 7)

Main bowel complaint
Duration of symptoms/trigger for onset
Usual bowel pattern   Any recent change?
Former bowel habit through adult life
Usual stool consistency:
    1. Lumps 2. Lumpy sausage 3. Cracked sausage 4. Soft smooth sausage
    5. Soft blobs 6. Fluffy, mushy 7. Watery, no pieces

Faecal incontinence: How often?   How much?
Urge to defaecate felt?
Urgency   Time can defer urgency for:
Urge incontinence: never/seldom/sometimes/frequently
Difficulty wiping: Yes ☐   No ☐   Sometimes ☐
Post-defaecation soiling: Yes ☐   No ☐   Sometimes ☐
Passive soiling: Yes ☐   No ☐   Sometimes ☐   Events causing?
Amount of flatus: Control of flatus: Good ☐   Variable ☐   Poor ☐
Ability to distinguish stool/flatus?   Yes ☐   No ☐
Abdominal pain relieved by defaecation?   Other pain?
Rectal bleeding?
Mucus?
Nocturnal bowel problems?

Evacuation difficulties?
Straining?
Sensation of incomplete evacuation?
Need to digitate anally, vaginally or to support the perineum?
Painful defaecation?

Bloating?
Sensation of rectal prolapse?
Pads used for faecal incontinence?
Bowel medication?   Other current medication
Past medical history (include psychological)
Toilet facilities
Able to communicate need to defaecate?
Assistance needed for toileting?
Physical or social difficulties with toilet access?
Previous bowel treatments and results
Obstetric history: parity   difficult deliveries or heavy babies?
Dietary influences on bowel function: fibre content of diet?
Smoker?
Weight/height/body mass index
Fluids (include caffeine)
Skin problems
Bladder problems
Effect on lifestyle/relationships; emotional/psychological effect

continued

> **Box 1 continued**
> **Examination**
> Visual inspection of anus
> Anal tone
> Ability to contract anal sphincter voluntarily
> Presence of stool in rectum
> Mental state examination
> Ability to toilet (include mobility, adjusting clothing, cleansing)

▪ coexistence of urinary incontinence

▪ medication review, including enquiry about:

   – laxative use

   – use of narcotic analgesia, antacids, calcium supplements and other constipating agents[11] (this is required because preventive care may need to be planned)

▪ other medical conditions (eg diabetes, neurological disease).[11]

Environment and psychological factors

▪ suitability of the toilet facilities and their accessibility (see Chapter 7)

▪ privacy and dignity, which older people consider one of the most important issues in bowel care

▪ if carers are needed to assist with toileting, their attitude towards this is crucial

▪ the effects of symptoms upon the individual and any carer(s) involved.

Physical examination

Physical examination should include:

▪ abdominal examination for presence of palpable faecal mass(es)

▪ anal inspection for evidence of soiling, rectal prolapse, peri-anal scarring, gaping anus and/or perineal descent

▪ digital anal examination to assess anal resting tone and squeeze; this correlates well with manometry measurements[12–14] and is reproducible when assessing the quality of contraction[15]

▪ digital rectal examination to determine whether there is faecal loading of the rectum or any abnormal rectal lesions – if the rectum is loaded, stool consistency should be assessed

▪ if rectal prolapse is suspected, the patient needs to be examined while straining on the toilet (examination in a supine position will often not demonstrate a prolapse)

∎ mobility and ability to self-toilet

∎ need for assistance with clothing and wiping

∎ cognitive assessment.

The Royal College of Nursing has issued clear guidelines on nurses performing digital rectal examination, stating that this is part of the nurse's role, provided that appropriate training has been given.[16] Trained nurses should be able to:

∎ inspect the anus for abnormalities

∎ detect the presence and consistency of stool in the rectum

∎ assess anal tone and the patient's ability to contract the anal sphincter voluntarily.

Bowel investigations

Abdominal radiograph

An empty rectum on digital rectal examination does not always exclude the diagnosis of constipation.[17,18] In this situation, an abdominal radiograph may help to determine whether faecal loading is present and to assess its extent. Faecal loading of the rectum with soft faeces was found in 47% of patients admitted to a geriatric medical assessment unit.[18] Patients with a large amount of faeces in the rectum did not always have colonic loading and vice versa. A transit study using radio-opaque markers may be more useful than a single abdominal X-ray.

Most radiologists in the UK and Europe[19] discourage overuse of this investigation. However, some clinicians consider it useful when evaluating the degree of bowel obstruction secondary to faecal impaction, in order to rule out acute complications of impaction such as sigmoid volvulus and stercoral perforation and to identify colonic dysmotility.[20-22]

Barium enema, colonoscopy, computed tomography

The symptoms of constipation, diarrhoea and/or faecal incontinence can be the presenting symptoms of colonic disease and may require investigation to exclude significant bowel pathology,[23] but not all incontinent patients will necessarily need such investigation. Profuse diarrhoea and incontinence are likely to occur during the bowel preparation for a barium enema and there is a high chance that older people will not retain the barium during the examination. Incontinence occurs during barium enema in 50% of patients, described as severe in 16%.[24] These patients may have endured an unpleasant preparation and test without any useful clinical information being obtained. Comparisons of colonoscopy versus barium enema in the investigation of possible colonic adenoma, carcinoma or angiodysplasia have suggested that colonoscopy is the investigation of choice in the elderly as it is more sensitive than barium enema.[25,26]

In a review of the use of these investigations Wolf *et al*[27] demonstrated that elderly and/or debilitated patients are often not capable of manoeuvring well enough on an X-ray table to give high-quality barium studies. Negative results may not therefore exclude the presence of disease, despite the unpleasant experience. Discomfort or pain during barium enema, which is related to incomplete bowel preparation, is more common in older people.[28] In some centres computed tomography scanning of the colon is now established as an alternative to barium enema in frail elderly patients.[29]

Bowel cancer

The incidence of lower gastrointestinal (GI) tumours (adenoma or carcinoma) increases with age. These typically present with a change in bowel habit, rectal bleeding, weight loss or large bowel obstruction. Any one or a combination of these symptoms should prompt examination of the lower GI tract. Traditionally, this has started with digital rectal examination followed – in the presence of rectal bleeding – by flexible sigmoidoscopy and double-contrast barium enema,[24] and then colonoscopy if the other investigations are negative.

Anorectal physiology tests

Anorectal physiology tests, including anal manometry, endoanal ultrasound, external sphincter electromyography and defaecating proctography, are not usually required in the routine clinical assessment of the frail older person. Even in surgical clinics they do not tend to alter the clinical examination conclusions or the management plan.[30]

EVIDENCE-BASED SUMMARY _____

(*Strength of evidence* [1]–[5]; see Appendix 1)

▪ Assessment should be multidisciplinary and multifactorial [2].

▪ A comprehensive assessment should include attention to bowel function, associated medical conditions, physical ability, cognitive function and access to toileting facilities [2].

WHAT WE DON'T KNOW

■ How can health professionals be encouraged to assess bowel function in frail older people?

■ What is the effect of a comprehensive assessment on planned care? Which factors are important to assess?

■ What is the reproducibility of the assessment?

■ Does assessment need to be done by a specialist or can a generalist do it equally well?

■ What training is needed to ensure that assessment skills are optimal?

■ What invasive bowel investigations are needed for frail older people with a change in bowel habit or rectal bleeding?

■ Is there a need for anorectal physiology tests in frail older people? What effect do they have on management?

■ What is the effect of bowel problems on the individual and carers (including psychosocial effects and quality of life)?

■ What are the costs of bowel problems? Do they differ when an intervention takes place?

References

1 Leigh RJ, Turnberg LA. Faecal incontinence: the unvoiced symptom. *Lancet* 1982;**i**:1349–51.

2 Edwards NI, Jones D. The prevalence of faecal incontinence in older people living at home. *Age Ageing* 2001;**30**:503–7.

3 Osterberg A, Graf W, Karlbom U, Pahlman L. Evaluation of a questionnaire in the assessment of patients with faecal incontinence and constipation. *Scand J Gastroenterol* 1996;**31**:575–80.

4 O'Keefe EA, Talley NJ, Tangalos EG, Zinsmeister AR. A bowel symptom questionnaire for the elderly. *J Gerontol* 1992;**47**:M116–21.

5 Morgan R, Spencer B, King D. Rectal examinations in elderly subjects: attitudes of patients and doctors. *Age Ageing* 1998;**27**:353–6.

6 Reilly WT, Talley NJ, Pemberton JH, Zinsmeister AR. Validation of a questionnaire to assess fecal incontinence and associated risk factors: Fecal Incontinence Questionnaire. *Dis Colon Rectum* 2000;**43**:146-53; discussion 153–4.

7 Norton C, Chelvanayagam S. A nursing assessment tool for adults with fecal incontinence. *J Wound Ostomy Continence Nurs* 2000;**27**:279–91.

8 Lewis SJ, Heaton KW. Stool form scale as a useful guide to intestinal transit time. *Scand J Gastroenterol* 1997;**32**:920–4.

9   Bliss DZ, Savik K, Jung H, Jensen L *et al.* Comparison of subjective classification of stool consistency and stool water content. *J Wound Ostomy Continence Nurs* 1999;**26**:137–41.

10 Engel AF, Kamm MA, Bartram CI, Nicholls RJ. Relationship of symptoms in faecal incontinence to specific sphincter abnormalities. *Int J Colorectal Dis* 1995;**10**:152–5.

11 Wrenn K. Fecal impaction. Review. *N Engl J Med* 1989;**321**:658–62.

12 Hallan RI, Marzouk DE, Waldron DJ, Womack NR, Williams NS. Comparison of digital and manometric assessment of anal sphincter function. *Br J Surg* 1989;**76**:973–5.

13 Felt-Bersma RJ, Klinkenberg-Knol EC, Meuwissen SG. Investigation of anorectal function. *Br J Surg* 1988;**75**:53–5.

14 Hill J, Corson RJ, Brandon H, Redford J *et al.* History and examination in the assessment of patients with idiopathic fecal incontinence. *Dis Colon Rectum* 1994;**37**:473–7.

15 Wyndaele JJ, Van Eetvelde B. Reproducibility of digital testing of the pelvic floor muscles in men. *Arch Phys Med Rehabil* 1996;**77**:1179–81.

16 Addison R, Smith M. *Digital Rectal Examination and Manual Removal of Faeces.* London: Royal College of Nursing, 2000.

17 Donald IP, Smith RG, Criukshank JG, Elton RA, Stoddart ME. A study of constipation in the elderly living at home. *Gerontology* 1985;**31**:112–8.

18 Smith RG, Lewis S. The relationship between digital rectal examination and abdominal radiographs in elderly patients. *Age Ageing* 1990;**19**:142–3.

19 European Commission in conjunction with the UK Royal College of Radiologists. *Referral Guidelines for Imaging.* Luxembourg: Office for Official Publications of the European Communities, 2001.

20 Harari D, Minaker KL. Megacolon in patients with chronic spinal cord injury. Review. *Spinal Cord* 2000;**38**:331–9.

21 McKay LF, Smith RG, Eastwood MA, Walsh SD, Cruickshank JG. An investigation of colonic function in the elderly. *Age Ageing* 1983;**12**:105–10.

22 Starreveld JS, Pols MA, Van Wijk HJ, Bogaard JW *et al.* The plain abdominal radiograph in the assessment of constipation. *Z Gastroenterol* 1990;**28**:335–8.

23 Boardman P, Nolan D. Computed tomography of the colon in elderly people. Single contrast barium study is adequate. *BMJ* 1994;**308**:1639.

24 Brewster NT, Grieve DC, Saunders JH. Double-contrast barium enema and flexible sigmoidoscopy for routine colonic investigation. *Br J Surg* 1994;**81**:445–7.

25 Irvine EJ, O'Connor J, Frost RA, Shorvon P *et al.* Prospective comparison of double contrast barium enema plus flexible sigmoidoscopy v colonoscopy in rectal bleeding: barium enema v colonoscopy in rectal bleeding. *Gut* 1988;**29**:1188–93.

26 Rex DK, Weddle RA, Lehman GA, Pound DC *et al.* Flexible sigmoidoscopy plus air contrast barium enema versus colonoscopy for suspected lower gastrointestinal bleeding. *Gastroenterology* 1990;**98**:855–61.

27 Wolf EL, Frager D, Beneventano T. Feasibility of double-contrast barium enema in the elderly. *Am J Roentgenol* 1985;**145**:47–8.

28 Steine S. Will it hurt, doctor? Factors predicting patients' experience of pain during double contrast examination of the colon. *BMJ* 1993;**307**:100.

29 Fink M, Freeman AH, Dixon AK, Coni NK. Computed tomography of the colon in elderly people. *BMJ* 1994;**308**:1018.

30 Keating JP, Stewart PJ, Eyers AA, Warner D, Bokey EL. Are special investigations of value in the management of patients with fecal incontinence? *Dis Colon Rectum* 1997;**40**:896–901.

5 | Treatment options for faecal incontinence

Christine Norton

Nurse Consultant (Bowel Control), St Mark's Hospital, North West London Hospitals NHS Trust, Harrow; Honorary Professor of Nursing, King's College, London

Management options

Research

Given the high prevalence of bowel problems in frail older people (Chapter 3), there has been remarkably little research on their management. Most major reviews of faecal incontinence fail to mention frail older people.[1–3] There are almost no high quality randomised trials in this area; the few studies that have been reported have often been small descriptive case-series. Most of the content of this chapter therefore relies on expert opinion or extrapolations from other patient populations. There is also a lack of validated outcome measures and no research on what outcomes are important to patients and what constitutes a clinically useful response to management.

In palliative care, there has been little assessment or documentation of bowel care. Carers have generally attempted to impose an arbitrary bowel regimen, without seeking information about the patient's previous bowel habits or preferences.[4]

Informed opinion

The importance of both a multidisciplinary assessment to identify and minimise impairments, disabilities and handicaps related to bowel dysfunction and of setting person-centred goals in line with desired post-rehabilitation lifestyle have been emphasised in relation to people with spinal cord injury.[5] The same principles should apply to frail older people. Any bowel schedule has to fit with other activities of the patient and any carer involved.

Bump and Norton[6] have suggested a model for the development of pelvic floor dysfunction which might be useful to conceptualise the myriad factors that can contribute to problems for each individual (Fig 1).

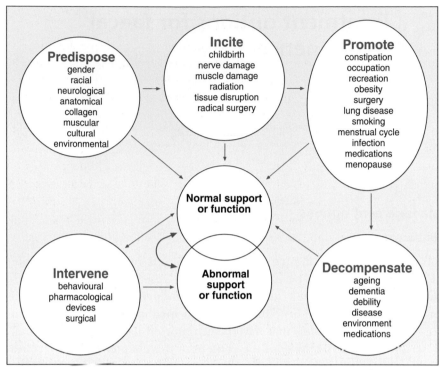

Fig 1. Model for the development of pelvic floor dysfunction in women.[6]

Many frail older people tread a fine dividing line between constipation and faecal incontinence, and care is needed that treatment for one of these does not precipitate the other. In practice, interventions will often be a combination of measures based on the individual's needs, as indicated by the comprehensive assessment outlined in Chapter 4.

Rectal evacuants, drugs and bowel training

Research

The two main approaches to management are the use of:

■ rectal evacuants to stimulate more effective evacuation of the bowel and establish a bowel pattern

■ anti-diarrhoeal agents to slow down an overactive bowel or to enable planned evacuation with rectal preparations.

There is no research base for either of these approaches in older people, but some work with other groups may be of relevance.[1]

Dunn and Galka[7] compared 'Therevac' micro-enemas (5 ml stimulant enemas) and bisacodyl suppositories in spinal injury patients and found that patients need over 45 minutes to respond to the suppositories. The micro-enemas reduced both digital stimulation time and evacuation time and, although much more expensive as medication, could potentially reduce carer time by up to one hour per day, with obvious cost savings. Two further randomised studies and one crossover study have found that the carrier is important for suppositories, with hydrogenated vegetable oil bisacodyl taking longer to work than polyethylene glycol-based bisacodyl. This is assumed to be the result of more rapid bioavailability as the former has to dissolve in body heat.[8,9] There is a theoretical risk of hyperphosphataemia from phosphate enemas in frail people with compromised electrolyte regulation, although this has been reported only in children.[10]

Compliance with prescribed medication is often poor. In a study of 114 rehabilitation patients, 66% were discharged taking bowel medication but a telephone interview one month later found that only 42% were still taking it.[11] It is unclear, though, whether this represents overprescribing and appropriate cessation at home or failure to comply with needed medication.

There is some evidence that suppositories are easier to insert and more effective if used blunt end first.[12] People with limited dexterity who need to use suppositories may find the Spinal Injuries Association suppository inserter helpful.

Some patients may effectively choose to stop spontaneous evacuation by using anti-diarrhoeal agents, and then plan evacuation at a convenient time by using suppositories or a micro-enema. Although not ideal, this regimen can at least give the patient an element of control and predictability to enable a reasonable quality of life. It has been found effective in a nursing home environment, even when staff compliance with prescribed regimens is not good (see below).[13]

A study in patients after a cerebrovascular accident found that a consistent elimination pattern was developed by a programme of daily digital rectal stimulation.[14] This was more effective than alternate day stimulation, with all but one of 25 patients achieving success. Patients with a right hemiplegia took longer to establish a pattern than those with a left hemiplegia, as did those with less mobility. Venn et al[15] found a morning bowel care regimen better than an evening one for establishing a bowel pattern after stroke, with the best results achieved if timing coincided with the premorbid bowel habit. There was no difference between suppositories given according to a schedule or only as needed, with 85% of patients achieving a pattern within one month. It is not known whether combining suppositories with digital stimulation might enhance the effect of the former.

In a nursing home population, frequency of defaecation and the number of continent stools was increased significantly in a trial of prompted voiding for urinary incontinence, although episodes of faecal incontinence were unchanged. The percentage of bowel actions passed continently rose from 18% before the programme to 45% afterwards.[16] The authors suggest that this incidental finding may relate to increased opportunity to sit on the toilet, together with improved mobility and fluid intake, and therefore that dependent individuals may increase bowel frequency simply by being able to access a toilet more frequently. This may have particular relevance for people with a urinary catheter who may seldom be offered use of the toilet.

Pharmacological approaches

Stool forming or bulking agents   Medication for faecal incontinence has usually involved either firming the stool with constipating agents such as loperamide or codeine phosphate, or stool bulking agents to give form to loose stool. Loperamide hydrochloride has been found to reduce faecal incontinence, improve stool consistency and reduce stool weight compared with placebo.[17] The authors suggested that stools might have been loose as a response to a weak anal sphincter. Loperamide oxide has a similar effect.[17] There is also some evidence that loperamide increases water absorption by slowing colonic transit and that, in an animal model, it decreases internal anal sphincter (IAS) relaxation in response to rectal distension[18] and increases mucosal fluid uptake.[19] After rectally infused saline, continence improved in 26 patients with chronic diarrhoea, and there was additionally a small increase in resting anal pressure.[20] Codeine phosphate is also effective for some patients.[21]

The safety and efficacy of these medications in frail older people have not been reported but, given that loose stool is highly associated with faecal incontinence, they have a potential role provided that bowel function is monitored to detect constipation.

Anal sphincter activity modification   A more recent pharmacological approach has been to modulate anal sphincter activity. Alpha-stimulant medication has been found to increase anal resting tone in healthy volunteers[22] and to improve incontinence in patients after formation of an ileo-anal pouch.[23] However, initial results in patients with 'idiopathic' incontinence have been disappointing.[24] This medication is contra-indicated in patients with cardiac problems and those with hypertension, which may limit the potential use in older people.

Other pharmacological approaches   Tobin and Brocklehurst[13] evaluated bowel care protocols in 52 patients living in residential homes who had faecal incontinence not associated with diarrhoea. Those found to be impacted (on rectal examination or a history of continuous faecal soiling) were given daily enemas until no further result was obtained. Other patients were presumed to have 'neurogenic' faecal incontinence and were treated with codeine phosphate 30–60 mg daily to stop spontaneous evacuation, and then given phosphate enemas twice weekly. The programme ran for two months and there was compliance with the protocol in two-thirds of patients. Among the compliant patients, 87% were no longer incontinent (94% with impaction, 75% neurogenic).

A different programme of daily Senokot and twice weekly enemas was tried in hospitalised elderly mentally ill patients without effect on faecal incontinence, although impaction improved. There was a huge variation in compliance between wards, ranging from 0% to 87%.[25]

There are oestrogen receptors in the external anal sphincter (EAS)[26] and hormone replacement therapy has been found of benefit in faecal incontinence in postmenopausal women in one uncontrolled study.[27] The role of hormone replacement in frail older women with bowel problems is not known.

Informed opinion

Many different interventions have been tried in the name of bowel training. Some authors suggest a package of care.[28] Scheduled attempts to defaecate will need to be timed if there is a loss of rectal sensation and the urge to defaecate is not felt. The bowel must first be cleared if necessary, followed by regulation of the stool consistency to a soft formed stool by diet or medication and a fluid intake of 30 ml/kg body weight per day. The recommended elements are:

▪ patient education about the importance of a prompt response to the call to stool

▪ using coffee to stimulate the gut

▪ capitalising on times likely for the gastro-colic response

▪ adopting a supported position on the toilet

▪ using a footstool to achieve a semisquat position.[28]

The bowel pattern should ideally be based on the premorbid bowel habit and may be daily or on alternate days. Where there is no spontaneous bowel action, this can be stimulated by digital stimulation, suppositories, a micro-enema or a tap water enema.[2,28,29]

Most authors extol the virtues of a high fibre diet, adequate fluid intake, as much exercise as feasible, and a regular toileting regimen to capitalise on the gastro-colic response. Where this fails to establish a habit, use of a suppository or digital stimulation is often advocated. In practice, many patients resort to evacuation by Valsalva or straining. However, this can eventually lead to problems with haemorrhoids or even rectal prolapse.

Biofeedback

Research

Faecal incontinence is a widely reported clinical indication for biofeedback. A recent review identified 46 studies (1,364 patients) published in English using biofeedback to treat adults complaining of faecal incontinence.[30] Only eight of the studies employed any form of control group. Of those studies with adequate data, 275 of 566 patients (49%) were said to be cured of symptoms of faecal incontinence following biofeedback therapy and 617 of 861 (72%) patients were reported to be cured or improved. Studies varied in the method of biofeedback used, criteria for success and the outcome measures used.

In the only study of the efficacy of biofeedback specifically in older patients,[31] 18 older people were initially treated for constipation as the presumed cause of faecal incontinence. Two became continent, two were excluded because of dementia and one because of absent rectal sensation. Half the remaining 13 patients were asked to perform 50 sphincter exercises per day for four weeks. These exercises did not improve sphincter function or continence compared with those who did not exercise, both groups having a reduction in episodes. All 13 then underwent biofeedback, which improved sphincter function and reduced incontinent episodes by at least 75% for 10 of them. This improvement was maintained in five at 12 months. Relapse was associated with debilitating diseases.

Many other studies have included a mixed group of consecutive patients presenting to a colorectal service with faecal incontinence, but it is not possible to extract information about frail older people.

Many different treatment modalities have been used in the name of 'biofeedback'. As described by the original authors, it was thought to be an operant conditioning therapy.[32] The aim was for the patient to learn to enhance the presumed reflex contraction of the EAS in response to a reflex relaxation of the IAS induced by stimulating the recto-anal inhibitory reflex by distension of a rectal balloon.[32] It has subsequently become evident that the EAS response is mostly a voluntary (if usually subconscious) response.[33] Later authors have recognised this and focused on training the patient to improve this voluntary response.

Biofeedback methods

No two studies have described exactly the same treatment as 'biofeedback'. Studies have used 1–28 sessions over two days to one year duration of therapy.

Electromyographic approach

An intra-anal electromyographic (EMG) sensor, an anal manometric probe (measuring intra-anal pressure) or peri-anal surface EMG electrodes are used to teach the patient how to exercise the anal sphincter, usually as a variation of pelvic floor muscle or Kegel exercises (more commonly used for the treatment of urinary incontinence).[34] In some cases this has been used simply to demonstrate correct isolation and use of an anal squeeze in response to rectal filling or an urge to defaecate. Others have devised a programme of home exercises, using the clinic biofeedback sessions to demonstrate correct technique and monitor progress in achievement. Early studies tended to focus on the peak muscle strength (squeeze increment),[35] while later workers have suggested that it is the overall muscle capacity (strength and endurance of the squeeze) that is important.[36,37]

Three-balloon system

A three-balloon system is used to 'train' the patient to identify correctly the stimulus of rectal distension and to respond without delay by immediate and forceful EAS contraction to counteract reflex inhibition of the IAS. Some have felt that sensory delay is an important factor in faecal incontinence, and that abolishing any delay in response to the sensation of distension is the crucial element in successful therapy.[38,39]

Rectal balloon

A rectal balloon is used to 'retrain' the sensory threshold, usually with the aim of enabling the patient to discriminate (and thus respond to) smaller rectal volumes. Improving (lowering) the threshold for sensing rectal distension has been found to be beneficial in reducing symptoms.[39] However, tolerance of larger volumes by the use of progressive distension and urge resistance is also reported.[40,41]

Other biofeedback approaches

Adjunctive therapies have included the use of electrical stimulation.[42,43] There are no reports of this in older people.

Biofeedback methods have also been used to treat constipation. Patients are taught to sit correctly on the toilet, relax the anal sphincter and co-ordinate abdominal effort while avoiding straining.[44] Over half of patients treated in this way achieve long-term benefit.[45] Although there are no reports specifically in frail older people, these techniques may be particularly appropriate to patients with neurological conditions that may predispose to paradoxical anal sphincter contraction on attempted defaecation, such as those with Parkinson's disease[46] or multiple sclerosis.[47]

Bowel washout regimens

Research

Bowel washouts are used much more frequently in Europe than in the UK. There is limited research on optimal regimens and techniques or on which fluids are the most effective. Gattuso et al[48] found that colostomy irrigation with water produced high-pressure propagated waves of colonic contraction and effective evacuation, without subsequent breakthrough, in volumes of 500 ml and above (but not at 250 ml). This work was not done with anal irrigation.

Some patients find it impossible to retain fluid instilled rectally. Using a catheter incorporating an inflatable balloon, Shandling and Gilmour[49] reported complete success with 40% of 112 children with spina bifida. Others are more cautious in their appraisal.[50] There are no studies of rectal washouts in frail older people.

Informed opinion

Clinical experience suggests that some patients with neurogenic bowel problems respond to rectal washout, often via a Foley catheter or enema balloon catheter if fluid is not easily retained,[51] but response is highly individual. To find the optimum for an individual, it is worth experimenting with volumes, temperatures and fluids, with or without addition of enemas.

Manual evacuation

Research

No study has examined the efficacy of this technique.

Informed opinion

A considerable controversy has arisen in nursing about the use of manual rectal evacuation and possible complications. There is limited research and no evidence of harmful effects. Undoubtedly there is a group of patients with little or no reflex activity in the lower colon (and so no ability to stimulate peristalsis), who have little alternative to planned manual evacuation done by either themselves or a carer or nurse. Some terminally ill patients, particularly those on heavy doses of opiate analgesia, may not respond to other evacuation methods. The majority of spinal cord injury patients need to use this regularly.[52]

The Royal College of Nursing[53] has reviewed manual evacuation and suggested a procedure and safety points. Their report clearly states for the first time that manual evacuation is a legitimate method of bowel management for carefully assessed and selected patients where other methods have failed.

Surgery

Research

Where pre-operative anal ultrasonography has demonstrated division of the EAS ring following trauma, caused for example by childbirth or previous anal fistula surgery, repair of the anal sphincter ring can achieve good short-term results[54] but longer-term results are less satisfactory.[55] Age does not preclude a successful outcome from sphincter repair surgery, but there is conflicting evidence whether outcome is worse[56] or better[57] in older people than in younger people.

In patients whose sphincter ring is intact but where the underlying aetiology is due to denervation, post-anal repair may be considered. In this procedure, the puborectalis muscle is plicated posterior to the anal canal, thus increasing the anorectal angle and increasing the length of the anal canal. However, long-term results are often unsatisfactory, even in younger patients.[58]

Where faecal incontinence is secondary to an external rectal prolapse, this will usually need repair which can be done via an anal approach in the frail patient. Prolapse is usually resolved, but it can recur and faecal incontinence may persist,[59] due either to sphincter damage or to neuropathy. Rectopexy for incomplete rectal prolapse does not seem to resolve incontinence.[60]

Informed opinion

There are no reports of surgery for faecal incontinence in frail older people. However, people whose physical disabilities have led to an inability to cope with the urgency consequent upon sphincter disruption may be considered for surgery.

Creation of a stoma may seem a drastic option but can make a dramatic contribution to quality of life for selected patients and their carers. If bowel function remains unpredictable and uncontrollable in the long term, it can be difficult to cope with. As discussed below, containment products are often unsatisfactory in enabling social continence for those with faecal incontinence. People with severe physical disabilities often find that inability to cope independently with toileting severely restricts their scope for activities, and carers may find a stoma easier to manage than incontinence. This option will need careful discussion and pre-operative counselling for all concerned.

General measures and advice

Research

Exercise has been found to increase propagated colonic contractions,[61,62] but may not be feasible for people with mobility difficulties. Abdominal massage in the direction of colonic peristalsis is often recommended and may be an alternative. In one pilot study of 12 immobile long-stay older people a 12-week programme of daily exercises and abdominal massage both significantly increased the number of bowel motions and decreased episodes of faecal incontinence and use of enemas. The use of laxatives virtually ceased – only one patient used one dose of laxative in the 12 weeks, whereas prior to therapy 11 had used laxatives daily.[63] The authors are cautious because of the lack of a control group, but these results are promising.

Nursing homes have been found not to have clear policies or protocols for managing faecal incontinence.[64] Accessibility and acceptability of toilet facilities or alternatives are likely to be crucial (see Chapter 7), but there is no research on this.

Informed opinion

It was suggested 40 years ago that staff in nursing homes tend to accept faecal incontinence as a normal part of nursing care, and that simple measures such as attention to diet, habit and posture, with active management for problems (eg suppositories, enemas, fluids, massage, improved mobility, clearing impaction) would promote bowel control.[65] Systematic evaluation of these simple measures has not yet occurred.

It is recommended that continence services address faecal as well as urinary incontinence.[66] Eleven benchmarks for high quality services have been proposed, including patient information and involvement, education for professionals and patients, and a physical and social environment which promotes continence.[67]

Patients with bowel problems often need considerable psychological support, together with teaching and information on the normal workings of the bowel (which most people have little idea about), and an understanding of what has gone wrong in their particular case. Knowledge about peristalsis, the gastro-colic reflex and the normal co-ordination of the IAS and EAS can enable planning and development of coping strategies. For example, many patients with urgency mistakenly contract their abdominal muscles in a desperate attempt to 'hang on' – in fact, this will exacerbate the tendency to urge incontinence if done when the IAS is reflexly relaxed upon rectal distension.[68] Others who move only with great effort find that incontinence can be precipitated if this exertion coincides with an urge to defaecate and a relaxed IAS. Explanation of the mechanism and advice to contract the EAS until the urge diminishes, and then go to the toilet can sometimes help, as can instruction on the best posture for effective defaecation.[69]

Fibre supplements

Many papers extol the virtues of a high fibre diet to regulate stool consistency and promote peristalsis. However, the evidence for efficacy of this is scant. One study added 40 g of wheat bran per day to the diet of spinal injury patients for three weeks. There was either no change or an increase in transit time, no change in stool weight and no decrease in the time taken for bowel evacuation.[70] It has been suggested that people with constipation may respond differently to fibre supplements from 'normals', and that fibre may even have a paradoxical effect of increasing transit times in an already sluggish bowel.[70] Fibre supplements can result in bloating and flatulence[61] and the need for an increased fluid intake, while some varieties such as ispaghula husk can be allergenic.[71] There is a risk of loss of iron, calcium and zinc with fibre supplements,[71] while unprocessed bran can interfere with vitamin and mineral absorption.

People with faecal incontinence not secondary to severe constipation may find it helpful to keep the stool firm and formed by moderating the fibre content of their diet. Immobile people are often found to have a colon loaded with soft stool which is more likely to leak than firm stool.[72] One-third of the constipated elderly have been found to have soft or liquid stool.[72] Fibre must be used with caution in immobile people as it has been found to increase the risk of faecal incontinence compared with placebo, with up to half of bed-bound people becoming incontinent with the addition of 10 g of wheat bran to the daily diet.[73] A soft impaction can be caused.[72] Fibre supplements are often said to be best avoided in people with dementia or neurological disease.[61]

Fluid intake

Increased fluid intake is often recommended for people with constipation. There is no evidence base for this, but stool consistency should improve in clinically dehydrated people and drinking itself may stimulate colonic propulsion.[74] Coffee seems to act as a gut stimulant for some people, particularly in the recto-sigmoid colon, with the response to caffeinated and decaffeinated drinks similar and more pronounced than drinking hot water.[74] Clinically, some patients with urgent defaection benefit from caffeine reduction,[68] while those who are constipated may use a drink of coffee to initiate defaecation.

Pressure sores

Faecal incontinence is associated with pressure sore development.[75] People at risk of pressure sore development, or who take a long time to evacuate, may benefit from an inflatable or gel toilet seat.

Managing intractable faecal incontinence

There are no perfect answers to the problem of coping with leakage from the bowel. It is difficult to find anything that reliably disguises bowel leakage and smell and very few products have been designed specifically for faecal leakage.

Pads and pants

No pad has been designed specifically for faecal incontinence. Most of the disposable pads used for urinary incontinence can be used for containment, but some people find them unnecessarily thick, bulky and not exactly the right shape to contain anal leakage. Many are available free of charge on the NHS via the district nurse or local continence nurse if there is a severe or regular problem.

Anal plug

An anal plug has been developed to help people with faecal incontinence. It is designed to be worn inside the rectum to plug the entrance to the anus from the inside. Some people find this uncomfortable or that it gives a constant feeling of needing to open the bowels. It has to be taken out before a bowel action, and so is not suitable for someone who needs to open the bowels very frequently. In one study, 11 of 14 patients (71%) withdrew the plug because of discomfort,[76] and in another only six of 20 patients could tolerate it.[77] This will obviously be less of a problem where anorectal sensation is impaired. The plug is worth trying, particularly for patients with passive soiling.

Skin care

Most people with faecal incontinence do not develop sore skin, but it can cause major distress for a minority. Loose stool, in particular, can rapidly excoriate the perianal skin and the coincidence of urinary incontinence may increase the risk of skin problems.[78] There has been little work on skin care in frail older people, although there are suggestions that proprietary skin cleansers may give greater skin protection than soap and water.[79]

Perineal cleaning can present a problem for someone with limited dexterity, and sometimes minor soiling is simply a result of ineffective wiping after defaecation. Moist toilet tissue is often more efficient than dry wiping. Toilet tongs or a bottom wiper can extend the reach of someone with limited shoulder or hand flexibility or strength. Where the toilet is next to the bath a showerhead may be usable. A portable bidet, which can be filled with warm water and will fit on any toilet, is also available.

Odour control

Meticulous personal hygiene and prompt disposal of soiled materials do not always ensure good odour control, and this can be the most embarrassing aspect of incontinence. Proprietary deodorants may be helpful. There are numerous other tips which can be tried to minimise the effect of odours.[68]

EVIDENCE-BASED SUMMARY ———————————————

(*Strength of evidence* [1]–[5]; see Appendix 1)

General measures

■ Exercise enhances bowel function [5].

■ An exercise programme with abdominal wall massage may improve bowel function in frail older people in long-term care settings [4].

■ Fibre can be used to alter stool consistency [2].

■ Additional fibre may exacerbate faecal incontinence in older people who are bed-bound, have dementia or other neurological causes for faecal incontinence [4].

- Coffee can be used as a gastro-colic stimulant to activate bowel function [5].
- Information for patients and carers helps in understanding and managing bowel care [5].
- Protocols for bowel management are required in long-term residential and nursing settings [5].

Rectal evacuants and toilet training

- Bowel control is improved by routines that increase access to the toilet, approximate to premorbid bowel routine and facilitate the gastro-colic effect of eating and activity [5].
- Bowel clearance with regular enemas re-established bowel continence in frail older people in residential care with faecal incontinence associated with a loaded rectum [4].
- Codeine phosphate with twice weekly enemas has been found to improve faecal incontinence in frail older people in residential care with faecal incontinence and an empty rectum [4].
- Daily senna with twice weekly enemas had no effect on faecal incontinence in hospitalised elderly mentally ill patients [4].
- Response time to the use of suppositories is slower than with micro-enemas and is related to the carrier constitution of the suppository (hydrogenated vegetable oil compared with polyethylene glycol) [1].
- Digital stimulation established consistent elimination in patients following cerebrovascular accident [4].

Biofeedback

- Biofeedback may have a role in improving faecal incontinence and constipation in frail older people, but this is unproven [4].

Bowel washout regimens

- Bowel washout regimens can be useful in clinical practice in achieving bowel clearance in older people [5].

Manual evacuation

- Manual evacuation is a legitimate method of bowel management in carefully selected and assessed patients [5].

Surgery

- Surgery in selected patients with appropriate indications (ie EAS tear, rectal prolapse) is effective in some older people in re-establishing bowel function [4].

▮ Stoma formation is an option in carefully selected older patients that can markedly enhance quality of life and improve bowel management [5].

Containment

▮ No pad is specifically designed for faecal incontinence [5].

▮ Anal plugs are frequently poorly tolerated but can be effective in helping contain faecal incontinence [4].

▮ Odour control can be the most embarrassing aspect of faecal incontinence. Methods exist to help with odour control [5].

Skin care

▮ Proprietary products may help in protecting skin from faecal incontinence [5].

▮ Physical disability reduces the ability to ensure skin protection after elimination [5].

▮ Assessment and appropriate management improve skin cleaning and protection [5].

▮ Inflatable or gel toilet seats reduce the risk of pressure breakdown of skin on defaecation [5].

WHAT WE DON'T KNOW

General measures

▮ What is the effect on continence of improving mobility? Studies have consistently found that poor mobility is related to faecal incontinence in the frail elderly.[76,81] It has been suggested that improving mobility is an approach to reducing the costs consequent upon incontinence.[82]

▮ What is the role of fibre supplements or fibre restriction?

▮ What is the efficacy of different sources and types of fibre?

▮ What is the role of abdominal massage?

▮ What are the roles of fluid amount, timing and type?

Management options

▮ There is no evidence on the appropriateness or responsiveness of any outcome measure or audit tool in this patient group.

- It is not known what outcomes are important to patients and their carers.
- There is little high quality evaluation of any single intervention for bowel care in frail older people.
- There are virtually no studies comparing different approaches to bowel care in frail older people.
- There are almost no studies in specific patient groups. For example, there are no studies of the treatment of faecal incontinence after stroke.[80]
- A multifactorial approach is often used in clinical practice, but the relative contribution of its components is unknown.
- There is a need to develop and evaluate stepwise algorithmic approaches.
- It is not known if a specialist health professional achieves better results than a generalist.

Rectal evacuants and bowel training

- What is the efficacy of rectal evacuants?
- Which is the most effective evacuant regimen?
- What is the efficacy of bowel training regimens?
- What toileting programmes are feasible and effective for improving bowel function in a nursing home setting?
- Which programme suits which patients?
- Is digital rectal stimulation effective and acceptable in this patient group?
- If stimulation is effective, there is a need to develop alternatives to the gloved finger.

Medication

- What is the role of anti-diarrhoeal medication in treating faecal incontinence associated with loose stool?
- What is the role of laxatives in treating or preventing incontinence associated with faecal loading?
- How can an acceptable balance be achieved between faecal incontinence and constipation?

Biofeedback

- Are biofeedback techniques acceptable and effective for treating faecal incontinence and constipation in frail older people?

▎ What is the role for biofeedback in treating paradoxical puborectalis contraction in the constipated frail older patient?

▎ What is the potential role of electrical stimulation for faecal incontinence in older patients?

▎ What is the role of sensory retraining in frail older people?

Bowel washout regimens

▎ Do bowel washout regimens work in frail older people?

▎ Is the technique acceptable to patients and carers?

▎ What is the risk of fluid balance and electrolyte disturbance in frail people?

▎ What regimen and volumes work best?

Manual evacuation

▎ What is the effect on anal sphincter function of prolonged use of manual evacuation?

Surgery

▎ Which patients might benefit from surgery?

▎ What are the outcomes in frail older people?

Managing intractable faecal incontinence

▎ What is the best skin care regimen for older people with faecal incontinence?

▎ Which is the most protective absorbent product?

▎ What is the role of the anal plug in this group?

References

1 Kamm MA. Faecal incontinence: clinical review. *BMJ* 1998;**316**:528–32.
2 Jorge JM, Wexner SD. Etiology and management of fecal incontinence. Review. *Dis Colon Rectum* 1993;**36**:77–97.
3 Madoff RD, Williams JG, Caushaj PF. Fecal incontinence. Review. *N Engl J Med* 1992;**326**:1002–7.
4 Cadd A, Keatinge D, Henssen M, O'Brien L *et al.* Assessment and documentation of bowel care management in palliative care: incorporating patient preferences into the care regimen. *J Clin Nurs* 2000;**9**:228–35.
5 Stiens SA, Bergman SB, Goetz LL. Neurogenic bowel dysfunction after spinal cord injury: clinical evaluation and rehabilitative management. Review. *Arch Phys Med Rehabil* 1997;**78**(3 Suppl):S86–102.
6 Bump RC, Norton PA. Epidemiology and natural history of pelvic floor dysfunction. Review. *Obstet Gynecol Clin North Am* 1998;**25**:723–46.

7   Dunn KL, Galka ML. A comparison of the effectiveness of Therevac SB and bisacodyl suppositories in SCI patients' bowel programs. *Rehabil Nurs* 1994;**19**: 334–8.

8   House JG, Stiens SA. Pharmacologically initiated defecation for persons with spinal cord injury: effectiveness of three agents. *Arch Phys Med Rehabil* 1997; **78**:1062–5.

9   Stiens SA. Reduction in bowel program duration with polyethylene glycol based bisacodyl suppositories. *Arch Phys Med Rehabil* 1995;**76**:674–7.

10 Hunter MF, Ashton MR, Griffiths DM, Ilangovan P *et al.* Hyperphosphataemia after enemas in childhood: prevention and treatment. *Arch Dis Child* 1993;**68**:233–4.

11 Graham C, Kunkle C. Do rehabilitation patients continue prescribed bowel medications after discharge? Review. *Rehabil Nurs* 1996;**21**:298–302.

12 And-el-Maeboud KH, el-Naggar T, el-Hawi EM. Rectal suppository – commonsense and mode of insertion. *Lancet* 1991;**338**:798–800.

13 Tobin GW, Brocklehurst JC. Faecal incontinence in residential homes for the elderly: prevalence, aetiology and management. *Age Ageing* 1986;**15**:41–6.

14 Munchiando JF, Kendall K. Comparison of the effectiveness of two bowel programs for CVA patients. *Rehabil Nurs* 1993;**18**:168–72.

15 Venn MR, Taft l, Carpentier B, Applebaugh G. The influence of timing and suppository use on efficiency and effectiveness of bowel training after a stroke. *Rehabil Nurs* 1992;**17**:116–20.

16 Ouslander JG, Simmons S, Schnelle J, Uman G, Fingold S. Effects of prompted voiding on fecal continence among nursing home residents. *J Am Geriatr Soc* 1996;**44**:424–8.

17 Sun WM, Read NW, Verlinden M. Effects of loperamide oxide in gastrointestinal transit time and anorectal function in patients with chronic diarrhoea and faecal incontinence. *Scand J Gastroenterol* 1997;**32**:34–8.

18 Rattan S, Culver PJ. Influence of loperamide on the internal anal sphincter in the opossum. *Gastroenterology* 1987;**93**:121–8.

19 Kamm MA. Functional disorders of the colon and anorectum. *Curr Opin Gastroenterol* 1995;**11**:9–15.

20 Read M, Read NW, Barber DC, Duthie HL. Effects of loperamide on anal sphincter function in patients complaining of chronic diarrhea with fecal incontinence and urgency. *Dig Dis Sci* 1982;**27**:807–14.

21 Barrett JA (ed). *Faecal Incontinence and Related Problems in the Older Adult.* London: Edward Arnold, 1993.

22 Carapeti EA, Kamm MA, Evans BK, Phillips RK. Topical phenylephrine increases anal sphincter resting pressure. *Br J Surg* 1999;**86**:267–70.

23 Carapeti EA, Kamm MA, Nicholls RJ, Phillips RK. Randomized, controlled trial of topical phenylephrine for fecal incontinence in patients after ileoanal pouch construction. *Dis Colon Rectum* 2000;**43**:1059–63.

24 Carapeti EA, Kamm MA, Phillips RK. Randomized controlled trial of topical phenylephrine in the treatment of faecal incontinence. *Br J Surg* 2000;**87**: 38–42.

25 Rands G, Malone-Lee J. Urinary and faecal incontinence in long stay wards for the mentally ill: prevalence and difficulties in management. *Health Trends* 1990;**22**:161–3.

26 Haadem K, Ling L, Ferno M, Graffner H. Estrogen receptors in the external anal sphincter. *Am J Obstet Gynecol* 1991;**164**:609–10.

27 Donnelly V, O'Connell PR, O'Herlihy C. The influence of oestrogen replacement on faecal incontinence in postmenopausal women. *Br J Obstet Gynaecol* 1997;**104**:311–5.

28 Doughty D. A physiologic approach to bowel training. *J Wound Ostomy Continence Nurs* 1996;**23**:46–56.

29 Jensen LL. Fecal incontinence: evaluation and treatment. Review. *J Wound Ostomy Continence Nurs* 1997;**24**:277–82.

30 Norton C, Kamm MA. Anal sphincter biofeedback and pelvic floor exercises for faecal incontinence in adults – a systematic review. Review. *Aliment Pharmacol Ther* 2001;**15**:1147–54.

31 Whitehead WE, Burgio KL, Engel BT. Biofeedback treatment of fecal incontinence in geriatric patients. *J Am Geriatr Soc* 1985;**33**:320–4.

32 Engel BT, Nikoomanesh P, Schuster MM. Operant conditioning of rectosphincteric responses in the treatment of fecal incontinence. *N Engl J Med* 1974;**290**:646–9.

33 Whitehead WE, Orr WC, Engel BT, Schuster MM. External anal sphincter response to rectal distension: learned response or reflex. *Psychophysiology* 1982;**19**:57–62.

34 Schussler B, Laycock J, Norton P, Stanton SL (eds). *Pelvic Floor Re-education: Principles and Practice.* London: Springer-Verlag, 1994.

35 MacLeod JH. Management of anal incontinence by biofeedback. *Gastroenterology* 1987;**93**:291–4.

36 Chiarioni G, Scattolini C, Bonfante F, Vantini I. Liquid stool incontinence with severe urgency: anorectal function and effective biofeedback treatment. *Gut* 1993;**34**:1576–80.

37 Patankar SK, Ferrara A, Larach SW, Williamson PR *et al.* Electromyographic assessment of biofeedback training for fecal incontinence and chronic constipation. *Dis Colon Rectum* 1997;**40**:907–11.

38 Buser WD, Miner PB Jr. Delayed rectal sensation with fecal incontinence. Successful treatment using anorectal manometry. *Gastroenterology* 1986;**91**:1186–91.

39 Miner PB, Donnelly TC, Read NW. Investigation of mode of action of biofeedback in treatment of fecal incontinence. *Dig Dis Sci* 1990;**35**:1291–8.

40 Oresland T, Fasth S, Hulten L, Nordgren S *et al.* Does balloon dilatation and anal sphincter training improve ileoanal-pouch function? *Int J Colorectal Dis* 1988;**3**:153–7.

41 Norton C, Kamm MA. Outcome of biofeedback for faecal incontinence. *Br J Surg* 1999;**86**:1159–63.

42 Fynes MM, Marshall K, Cassidy M, Behan M *et al.* A prospective, randomized study comparing the effect of augmented biofeedback with sensory biofeedback alone on fecal incontinence after obstetric trauma. *Dis Colon Rectum* 1999;**42**:753–8; discussion 758–61.

43 Sander P, Bjarnesen J, Mouritsen L, Fuglsang-Frederiksen A. Anal incontinence after obstetric third-/fourth-degree laceration. One-year follow-up after pelvic floor exercises. *Int Urogynecol J Pelvic Floor Dysfunct* 1999;**10**:177–81.

44 Storrie JB. Biofeedback: a first-line treatment for idiopathic constipation. Review. *Br J Nurs* 1997;**6**:152–8.

45 Chiotakakou-Faliakou E, Kamm MA, Roy AJ, Storrie JB, Turner IC. Biofeedback provides long-term benefit for patients with intractable, slow and normal transit constipation. *Gut* 1998;**42**:517–21.

46 Edwards LL, Quigley EM, Harned RK, Hofman R, Pfeiffer RF. Characterization of swallowing and defecation in Parkinson's disease. *Am J Gastroenterol* 1994;**89**:15–25.

47 Chia YW, Gill KP, Jameson JS, Forti AD *et al.* Paradoxical puborectalis contraction is a feature of constipation in patients with multiple sclerosis. *J Neurol Neurosurg Psychiatry* 1996;**60**:31–5.

48 Gattuso JM, Kamm MA, Myers C, Saunders B, Roy A. Effect of different infusion regimens on colonic motility and efficacy of colostomy irrigation. *Br J Surg* 1996;**83**:1459–62.

49 Shandling B, Gilmour RF. The enema continence catheter in spina bifida: successful bowel management. *J Pediatr Surg* 1987;**22**:271–3.

50 Liptak GS, Revell GM. Management of bowel dysfunction in children with spinal cord disease or injury by means of the enema continence catheter. *J Pediatr* 1992;**120**:190–4.

51 Christensen P, Kvitzau B, Krogh K, Buntzen S, Laurberg S. Neurogenic colo-rectal dysfunction – use of new antegrade and retrograde colonic wash-out methods. *Spinal Cord* 2000;**38**:255–61.

52 Glickman S, Kamm MA. Bowel dysfunction in spinal-cord-injury patients. *Lancet* 1996;**347**:1651–3.

53 Addison R, Smith M. *Digital Rectal Examination and Manual Removal of Faeces.* London: Royal College of Nursing, 2000.

54 Engel AF, Kamm MA, Sultan AH, Bartram CI, Nicholls RJ. Anterior anal sphincter repair in patients with obstetric trauma. *Br J Surg* 1994;**81**:1231–4.

55 Malouf A, Norton CS, Engels AF, Nicholls RJ, Kamm MA. Long-term results of overlapping anterior anal-sphincter repair for obstetric trauma. *Lancet* 2000;**355**:260–5.

56 Rasmussen OO, Puggaard L, Christiansen J. Anal sphincter repair in patients with obstetric trauma: age affects outcome. *Dis Colon Rectum* 1999;**42**:193–5.

57 Young CJ, Mathur MN, Eyers AA, Solomon MJ. Successful overlapping anal sphincter repair: relationship to patient age, neuropathy, and colostomy formation. *Dis Colon Rectum* 1998;**41**:344–9.

58 Jameson JS, Speakman CT, Darzi A, Chia YW, Henry MM. Audit of postanal repair in the treatment of fecal incontinence. *Dis Colon Rectum* 1994;**37**: 369–72.

59 Hool GR, Hull TL, Fazio VW. Surgical treatment of recurrent complete rectal prolapse: a thirty-year experience. *Dis Colon Rectum* 1997;**40**:270–2.

60 Briel JW, Schouten WR, Boerma MO. Long-term results of suture rectopexy in patients with fecal incontinence associated with incomplete rectal prolapse. *Dis Colon Rectum* 1997;**40**:1228–32.

61 Wald A. Constipation and fecal incontinence in the elderly. Review. *Semin Gastrointest Dis* 1994;**5**:179–88.

62 Crowell MD, Bassotti G, Cheskin LJ, Schuster MM, Whitehead WE. Method for prolonged ambulatory monitoring of high-amplitude propagated contractions from the colon. *Am J Physiol* 1991;**261**:G263–8.

63 Resende TL, Brocklehurst JC, O'Neill PA. A pilot study on the effect of exercise and abdominal massage on bowel habit in continuing care patients. *Clin Rehabil* 1993;**7**:204–9.

64 Thomas TM, Ruff C, Karran O, Mellows S, Meade TW. Study of the prevalence and management of patients with faecal incontinence in old people's homes. *Community Med* 1987;**9**:232–7.

65 Saxon J. Techniques for bowel and bladder training. *Am J Nurs* 1962;**62**:69–71.

66 Department of Health. *Good Practice in Continence Services.* PL/CMO/2000/2. London. NHS Executive, 2000.

67 NHS Executive. *The Essence of Care: Continence and Bladder and Bowel Care.* Leeds: NHS Executive, 2001:98.

68 Norton C, Kamm MA. *Bowel Control – Information and Practical Advice.* Beaconsfield: Beaconsfield Publishers, 1999.

69 Markwell S, Sapsford R. Physiotherapy management of obstructed defaecation. *Aust J Physiother* 1995;**41**:279–83.

70 Cameron K, Nyulasi I, Collier GR, Brown DJ. Assessment of the effect of

increased dietary fibre intake on bowel function in patients with spinal cord injury. *Spinal Cord* 1996;**34**:277–83.

71 Gattuso JM, Kamm MA. Review article: the management of constipation in adults. Review. *Aliment Pharmacol Ther* 1993;**7**:487–500.

72 Barrett JA. Effects of wheat bran on stool size. *BMJ* 1988;**296**:1127–8.

73 Ardron ME, Main AN. Management of constipation. *BMJ* 1990;**300**:1400.

74 Brown SR, Cann PA, Read NW. Effect of coffee on distal colon function. *Gut* 1990;**31**:450–3.

75 Brocklehurst JC, Andrews K, Richards B, Laycock PJ. Incidence and correlates of incontinence in stroke patients. *J Am Geriatr Soc* 1985;**33**:540–2.

76 Christiansen J, Roed-Petersen K. Clinical assessment of the anal continence plug. *Dis Colon Rectum* 1993;**36**:740–2.

77 Norton C, Kamm MA. Anal plug for faecal incontinence. *Colorectal Dis* 2001;**3**: 323–7.

78 Schnelle JF, Adamson GM, Cruise PA, al-Samarrai N *et al*. Skin disorders and moisture in incontinent nursing home residents: intervention implications. *J Am Geriatr Soc* 1997;**45**:1182–8.

79 Cooper P, Gray D. Comparison of two skin care regimes for incontinence. *Br J Nursing* 2001;**10**:S6–20.

80 Brittain KR, Peet SM, Castleden CM. Stroke and incontinence. Review. *Stroke* 1998;**29**:524–8.

81 Chassagne P, Landrin I, Neveu C, Czernichow P *et al*. Fecal incontinence in the institutionalized elderly: incidence, risk factors, and prognosis. *Am J Med* 1999;**106**:185–90.

82 Borrie MJ, Bawden ME, Kartha AS, Kerr PS. A nurse/physician continence clinic triage approach for urinary incontinence: a 25 week randomised trial. *Neurourol Urodyn* 1992;**11**:364–5.

6 | The use and abuse of laxatives in older people

Anton Emmanuel

Senior Lecturer and Consultant Gastroenterologist,
St Mark's Hospital, London

Medications predisposing towards constipation

If an older person develops the onset or sudden worsening of the symptom of constipation, clinical evaluation should in the first instance be directed towards excluding a treatable organic cause. Colorectal cancer, hypothyroidism or other metabolic disorder and neurological disorders are amongst the commoner conditions to be excluded by appropriate clinical assessment and examination.

The corollary is that patients with chronic symptoms should not be subjected to repeated, time-consuming and unnecessary investigation. Most patients with chronic constipation are on multiple other medications for coexisting illness.[1] Such polypharmacy is most prevalent in long-term care patients.[2] For obvious methodological reasons, the literature lacks studies directly linking specific agents with the development of constipation. Nonetheless, a large amount of clinical experience implicates several classes of drug as especially likely to provoke symptoms of constipation. Furthermore, the nature of the reporting process for drug side effects is likely substantially to under-report drugs causing constipation.[3]

Certain medications are well recognised as being constipating, notably opiates and agents with anticholinergic properties. Many other agents with a strong constipating action are frequently prescribed in older people. A list of well-recognised constipating agents is shown in Box 1. Wherever possible, these drugs should be discontinued and other non-constipating agents used.

Laxative misuse

Annual expenditure on laxatives in England is £43 million, more even than is spent on antihypertensives.[4] One-quarter of regular laxative-using older subjects do not consider themselves to be constipated.[5] Over-the-counter (OTC) laxatives are used by approximately one-quarter of older people.[6] This high consumption reflects both the widespread

Box 1. Potentially constipating drugs		
Opiates		
Anticholinergic drugs	Antidepressants	
	Antipsychotics	
	Anti-parkinsonians	
	Antispasmodics	
	Antihistamines	
Diuretics		
Oral iron supplements		
Sympathomimetics	Ephedrine	
	Phenylephrine	
	Terbutaline	
Antacids	Aluminium-containing agents	
Antihypertensives	Calcium-channel antagonists	
	Clonidine	
	Angiotensin-converting enzyme inhibitors	
Non-steroidal anti-inflammatory drugs		

availability of OTC laxatives[7] and the widely held misconception amongst older people of the dangers of 'auto intoxication' without a daily bowel action.[8,9] Once this is recognised, laxative misuse must be discouraged as the first step of management.

The problem of laxative misuse is not, however, confined to the community. About half of all older institutionalised patients are taking at least one laxative.[10,11] Institutionalised patients are most likely to be prescribed stool softeners, in contrast to the older population in the community amongst whom bulking agents are the most commonly consumed laxatives.

Preventive treatment

Before discussing the laxatives available for managing chronic idiopathic constipation in older people, it is important briefly to consider the literature on preventive and non-laxative management including the need to avoid laxative misuse. Even when laxatives are needed to treat a patient, these non-pharmacological measures should be implemented and maintained.

Non-pharmacological treatment

Once the diagnosis of idiopathic constipation has been confirmed, the need for disimpaction should be considered.[12] Thereafter, patient education is the cornerstone of management. Improving dietary habits, optimising mobility, and education about toileting behaviour should be undertaken.[13] Briefly, patients need to be instructed to allow time for a bowel action at times when gut motility is greatest, namely on rising and after meals. Healthcare professionals need to pay attention to treating underlying psychiatric, neurological and metabolic abnormalities.[14,15]

Although fibre supplementation does not accelerate whole gut transit in older subjects,[16] it has been shown in non-randomised studies to reduce laxative consumption and improve bowel frequency.[17-21] Coarse bran, though less palatable, is more effective than refined fibre, but is associated with the development of abdominal pain and flatulence.[22] It is unknown whether the results found in the studies[17-21] are due to an effect of the fibre supplementation itself or to increased fluid intake. However, there is no evidence that dehydration in older people results in constipation.[23]

Laxative and enema use in older people

Quality of research

Reported clinical trials of laxatives and enemas tend not to have been of the highest quality. The trials are limited from the outset by the variability of definition. There is also variability of reported outcome parameters (bowel frequency, stool consistency, abdominal pain, 'overall symptoms', need for additional laxatives or enemas). This is added to by the variable recording of these measurement outcomes, some studies relying on self-reported symptoms and others using health professional-reported bowel symptoms, both of which are known to be potentially inaccurate and unreliable.[24] Many of the trials failed to document fibre and fluid intake amongst the subjects – or indeed any of the other possible confounding variables. Additionally, some trials used combination laxatives containing more than one class of agent, thereby limiting the conclusions that can be drawn about the different classes of agent. In many cases the incidence of adverse events was not recorded. Treatment duration for most trials was four weeks or less; given that most patients have chronic symptoms, this limits the recommendations that can be extrapolated from these studies. Most of the studies were not double-blind and lacked sufficient numbers to generate statistical power. With a high placebo response, as seen in most functional gastrointestinal disorders,[25] studies comparing laxatives need to be large enough to detect clinically significant differences.

Laxative trials carried out in the general adult population will not be considered in this review because there are insufficient data about the older subjects included in those trials to allow analysis.[26-28]

Randomised placebo-controlled trials

Bulking agents

Two double-blind[29,30] and two non-blinded studies[31,32] have compared bulking agents with placebo or normal diet. They were all small studies (total number of patients 83, range 10–51). None showed any differences in bowel frequency, and the only statistically significant difference reported was in stool consistency in one study.[29] Typical of trials with bulking agents, there was a near one-third dropout rate, limiting the statistical power. The Cheskin *et al* study[32] was the only one in a primary care setting.

Stool softening agents

In a double-blind, placebo-controlled trial of docusate sodium in 40 patients, Hyland and Foran[33] reported an improvement in overall symptom burden with active treatment. There were, however, no changes in stool frequency or consistency and the study had a very high (60%) dropout rate.

Osmotic agents

Two double-blind, placebo-controlled trials of either lactulose or lactitol[34,35] in the literature and one non-blinded study of lactulose[36] showed a consistent improvement in stool frequency, consistency and overall symptoms in favour of osmotic laxatives. Sample sizes were comparatively large (43–103 patients) in these studies and dropout rates low.

Stimulant agents

Stern[37] reported a double-blind, placebo-controlled trial of prucara in 25 institutionalised patients, showing improved stool consistency and control of defaecation. Using a complicated, non-blinded study design Marchesi[38] compared cascara and boldo given jointly (a South American bark derivative) with placebo in 14 patients. There was a statistically improved stool frequency and consistency.

Randomised controlled trials comparing different laxatives in the same class

Bulking agents

Chokhavatia *et al*[39] conducted a non-blinded comparison in 42 outpatients of three weeks' treatment with calcium polycarbophil or psyllium. There was no difference between the agents for stool frequency, consistency or need to strain. Calcium polycarbophil, however, was better tolerated in terms of flatulence.

Osmotic agents

There are two studies in the literature comparing lactulose with a cheaper osmotic agent, either sorbitol[40] or lactitol,[41] both in patients in long-term care facilities. The larger study (n = 60) reported a statistically increased weekly bowel frequency with lactitol. The clinical significance of this small difference in mean weekly bowel frequency (5.5 vs 4.9) is uncertain, especially since the study was non-blinded. Both studies reported that the medications were well tolerated. The study comparing lactulose and sorbitol[40] undertook a pricing assessment and found that sorbitol was more cost-effective.

Stimulant agents

Marchesi[38] reported a three-limb, non-blinded study of 14 hospitalised older patients, comparing a cascara/boldo preparation with two doses of inositol/vitamin B12. No differences in bowel frequency were reported between the three treatment groups.

Randomised controlled trials comparing laxatives from different classes

There are six trials in the literature comparing the efficacy and tolerability of different laxative classes in older people. There is great variety in the choice of agents (whether single or in combination), trial sizes (20–85 patients) and design, so the studies will be discussed separately. All the studies were conducted in either hospitalised or institutionalised patients, with no reports in the primary care setting.

1 A three-week trial comparing dorbanex with sodium picosulphate in 40 institutionalised patients found that dorbanex, which has both softening and stimulant actions, was better tolerated than picosulphate (a stimulant alone) and more effective in terms of stool frequency and consistency.[42]

2 Fain *et al*[43] conducted a non-blinded comparison of a softening agent (dioctyl calcium sulphosuccinate) with a stimulant (dioctyl sodium sulphosuccinate) in 47 institutionalised patients. They reported the slightly surprising finding that the softener did not change stool consistency compared with the stimulant, but did increase bowel frequency.

3 Pers and Pers[44] compared two similar agents, agiolax and lunelax, in a non-blinded study of 20 hospitalised older patients. Both drugs are a combination of a bulking and stimulating agent and were equally well tolerated. Lunelax was reported as significantly more effective than agiolax in terms of improving bowel frequency.

4 A bulking agent (laxamucil) and an osmotic agent (magnesium hydroxide) were compared in 64 institutionalised older patients in a non-blinded study.[45] The results showed an advantage for magnesium hydroxide in terms of improving stool frequency and consistency, whilst reducing other laxative consumption.

5 A large, double-blind study of 85 institutionalised patients compared an osmotic agent, lactulose, with agiolax.[46] Agiolax significantly improved stool frequency and consistency compared with lactulose. This study also included assessment of cost-effectiveness expressed in terms of a 'cost-per-stool' for each treatment and found that the comparative figures for lactulose and agiolax were £0.40 and £0.10, respectively.

6 Kinnunen *et al*[47] compared the same agents in a smaller, non-blinded study in 20 patients in a similar setting. Agiolax was again reported as superior to lactulose in terms of increasing stool frequency and reducing consumption of other laxatives, but it was more likely to result in loose stools, raising concerns about faecal continence.

Enemas and faecal disimpaction

Regular phosphate enemas have been reported as an equally effective alternative to osmotic or stimulant agents in treating older institution-alised patients with constipation.[24] Used in an as-required fashion, enemas also have a place in the management of patients with rectal impaction.[24] Polyethylene glycol, an osmotic laxative, has been studied in the management of faecal impaction.[48] Two days' oral treatment with Movicol®, a potent polyethylene glycol drug, complemented by daily phosphate enemas until resolution, has been found effective in treating recto-sigmoid impaction.[48] A practical approach to the management of older patients with faecal impaction is presented in Fig 1.

Although never subjected to formal clinical trial, enemas and supposi-tories are widely recognised as helpful in patients whose symptoms of constipation primarily relate to difficulty with rectal evacuation.

Conclusions regarding studies of laxative use in older people

The research base presented is derived almost exclusively from studies of

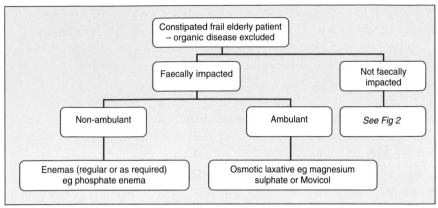

Fig 1. An approach to treating faecal disimpaction in the frail elderly.

patients in hospital or institutional care. Extrapolation to draw conclusions for older patients in the community would not be appropriate.[49] The relative lack of methodologically sound trials for treatment of constipation in older people is in contrast to the situation in the general adult population (reviewed by Tramonte *et al*).[50] Older people are the main consumers of laxatives in the community,[6,51] so this double lack of data – both from older people in general and from the primary care setting, in particular – is an important research area to address.

In placebo-controlled studies, only the osmotic laxatives (and to a lesser extent the stimulant agents) showed a significant improvement in bowel function in older subjects complaining of constipation. In non-placebo-controlled studies, there is evidence supporting a beneficial role with all laxative classes. Furthermore, in contrast to the placebo-controlled studies, two trials have reported an advantage of a combined preparation of bulking agent and stimulant over an osmotic laxative. On balance, given the low methodological quality of the available data, it is difficult to be dogmatic about treatment recommendations. A pragmatic evidence-based approach to constipation in the non-faecally impacted older person is suggested in Fig 2.

The cost per month of the most commonly used agents of each class is listed in Box 2. In view of the lack of high quality research data, there is no evidence base to support continued prescribing of the more expensive laxatives.

EVIDENCE-BASED SUMMARY ―――――――――――――――――――

(*Strength of evidence* [1]–[5]; see Appendix 1)

▪ In placebo-controlled trials only osmotic laxatives (and to a lesser

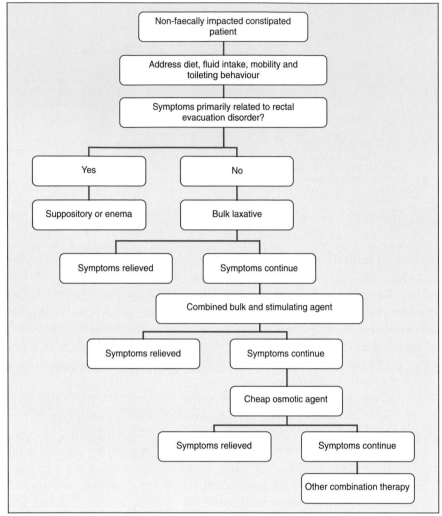

Fig 2. An approach to treating constipation in frail, non-faecally impacted older people.

extent) stimulating agents showed a significant improvement in bowel function in older people [1].

▪ In comparisons between agents, combination treatment with bulking and stimulating agents were more effective than osmotic laxatives alone [2].

▪ There is no evidence base to support continued prescribing of expensive laxatives [2].

▪ In older people in long-term care settings:

Box 2. Cost per month of each class of laxative (as used in standard clinical dose, based on British National Formulary pricing September 2000)

Class of laxative	Drug	Dose	Cost per month (£)
Bulking agents	Fybogel	1 sachet bd	4.24
	Normacol	1 sachet bd	4.65
Softening agents	Docusate sodium	100 mg tds	5.04
Osmotic agents	Magnesium sulphate	10 g od	0.99
	Lactitol	20 g od	6.00
	Lactulose	30 ml bd	9.47
	Macrogols (Movicol®)	2 sachets bd	26.10
Stimulant agents	Senna	3 tablets od	1.35
	Bisacodyl	10 mg od	1.86
	Sodium picosulfate	10 ml od	5.55
	Co-danthramer	2 capsules od	12.82
Combined bulking and stimulant agents	Manevac	4 g bd	4.07
Suppositories and enemas	Glycerol	1 suppository bd	4.60
	Fleet enema	(3 x per week)	6.10
	Phosphate enema	(3 x per week)	

od = once per day; bd = twice per day; tds = three times per week.

– Stimulating and bulking agent combined were more effective than stimulating agent alone on stool frequency and consistency [4].

– Osmotic agents were more effective than bulking agents for stool consistency and frequency [4].

– Stimulating agents improve stool frequency and consistency compared with osmotic agents [4].

– Phosphate enemas are as effective as osmotic and stimulant agents in treating constipation [4].

– Suppositories and enemas are helpful in treating patients whose symptoms primarily relate to a rectal evacuation disorder [5].

WHAT WE DON'T KNOW

▌ Laxative studies to date have employed crude end-points such as stool frequency or consistency. More appropriate and precise end-points are required in assessing laxative use. This is especially important in view of the well recognised abnormal beliefs and behaviour regarding gut function expressed by the elderly.[9,13]

- There is a need for improved outcome measures which have a direct bearing on the patients' subjective feelings about their condition.
- There is a need to explore issues of quality of life in the elderly – similar to the research undertaken in the general adult population on the impact of chronic idiopathic constipation.[52]
- What are the effective management regimens for constipation in the elderly population living in the community? Such studies should encompass non-pharmacological interventions as well as appropriate laxative treatment.
- For hospitalised or institutionalised patients with constipation, there is a need for a large-scale study of a stepped care approach to treatment along the lines outlined above.
- The potential role for the new gut prokinetics, the serotonin agonists and antagonists[53] in treating constipation in the frail elderly needs to be addressed.

References

1. Whitehead WE, Drinkwater D, Cheskin LJ, Heller BR, Schuster MM. Constipation in the elderly living at home. Definition, prevalence, and relationship to lifestyle and health status. *J Am Geriatr Soc* 1989;**37**:423–9.

2. Gurwitz JH, Soumerai SB, Avorn J. Improving medication prescribing and utilization in the nursing home. Review. *J Am Geriatr Soc* 1990;**38**:542–52.

3. Tedesco FJ, DiPiro JT. Laxative use in constipation. Review. American College of Gastroenterology's Committee on FDA-related matters. *Am J Gastroenterol* 1985;**80**:303–9.

4. Petticrew M, Watt I, Brand M. What's the 'best buy' for treatment of constipation? Results of a systematic review of the efficacy and comparative efficacy of laxatives in the elderly. Review. *Br J Gen Pract* 1999;**49**:387–93.

5. Connell AM, Hilton C, Irvin G, Lennard-Jones JE, Misiewicz JJ. Variation in bowel habit in two population samples. *BMJ* 1965;**2**:1095–7.

6. Stoehr GP, Ganguli M, Seaberg EC, Echemont DA, Belle S. Over-the-counter medication use in an older rural community: the MoVIES project. *J Am Geriatr Soc* 1997;**45**:158–65.

7. Johnson RE, Vollner WM. Comparing sources of drug data about the elderly. *J Am Geriatr Soc* 1991;**39**:1079–84.

8. Moore-Gillon V. Constipation: what does the patient mean? *J R Soc Med* 1984;**77**:108–10.

9. Whorton J. Civilisation and the colon: constipation as the 'disease of diseases'. *BMJ* 2000;**321**:1586–9.

10. Lamy PP, Krug BH. Review of laxative utilization in a skilled nursing facility. *J Am Geriatr Soc* 1978;**26**:544–9.

11. Harari D, Gurwitz JH, Avorn J, Choodnovskiy I, Minaker KL. Constipation: assessment and management in an institutionalized elderly population. *J Am Geriatr Soc* 1994;**42**:947–52.

12   Wrenn K. Fecal impaction. Review. *N Engl J Med* 1989;**321**:658–62.
13   Castle SC. Constipation: endemic in the elderly? Gerontopathology, evaluation and management. *Med Clin North Am* 1989;**73**:1497–509.
14   Garvey M, Noyes R Jr, Yates W. Frequency of constipation in major depression: relationship to other clinical variables. *Psychosomatics* 1990;**31**:204–6.
15   Jost WH, Schimrigk K. Constipation in Parkinson's disease. *Klin Wochenschr* 1991;**69**:906–9.
16   Muller-Lissner SA. Effect of wheat bran on the weight of stool and gastro-intestinal transit time: a meta-analysis. *BMJ* 1988;**296**;615–7.
17   Hull C, Greco RS, Brooks DL. Alleviation of constipation in the elderly by dietary fiber supplementation. *J Am Geriatr Soc* 1980;**28**:410–4.
18   Pringle R, Pennington MJ, Pennington CR, Ritchie RT. A study of the influence of a fibre biscuit on bowel function in the elderly. *Age Ageing* 1984; **13**:175–8.
19   Valle-Jones JC. An open study of oat bran biscuits ('Lejfibre') in the treatment of constipation in the elderly. *Curr Med Res Opin* 1985;**9**:716–20.
20   Hope AK, Down EC. Dietary fibre and fluid in the control of constipation in a nursing home population. *Med J Aust* 1986;**144**:306–7.
21   Egger G, Wolfenden K, Pares J, Mowbray G. 'Bread: it's a great way to go'. Increasing bread consumption decreases laxative sales in an elderly community. *Med J Aus* 1991;**155**:820–1.
22   Taylor R. Controversies in therapeutics: management of constipation: high fibre diets work. *BMJ* 1990;**300**:1063–4.
23   Harari D, Gurwitz JH, Minaker KL. Constipation in the elderly. Review. *J Am Geriatr Soc* 1993;**41**:1130–40.
24   Brocklehurst JC, Kirkland JL, Martin J, Ashford J. Constipation in long-stay elderly patients: its treatment and prevention by lactulose, polaxalkol-dihydroxyanthroquinolone and phosphate enemas. *Gerontology* 1983;**29**: 181–4.
25   Spiller RC. Problems and challenges in the design of irritable bowel syndrome clinical trials: experience from published trials. Review. *Am J Med* 1999;**107**:91S–7S.
26   Connolly P, Hughes IW, Ryan G. Comparison of 'Duphulac' and 'irritant' laxatives during and after treatment of chronic constipation: a preliminary study. *Curr Med Res Opin* 1985;**2**:620–5.
27   Odes HS, Madar Z. A double-blind trial of celandin, aloevera and psyllium laxative preparation in adult patients with constipation. *Digestion* 1991;**49**: 65–71.
28   Rouse M, Chapman N, Mahapatra M, Grillage M *et al.* An open, randomised, parallel group study of lactulose versus ispaghula in the treatment of chronic constipation in adults. *Br J Clin Pract* 1991;**45**:28–30.
29   Ewerth S, Ahlberg J, Holmstrom B, Persson U, Uden R. Influence on symptoms and transit-time of Vi-SiblinR in diverticular disease. *Acta Chir Scand Suppl* 1980;**500**:49–50.
30   Rajala SA, Salminen SJ, Seppanen JH, Vapaatalo H. Treatment of chronic constipation with lactitol sweetened yoghurt supplemented with guar gum and wheat bran in elderly hospital in-patients. *Compr Gerontol [A]* 1988;**2**:83–6.
31   Finlay M. The use of dietary fibre in a long-stay geriatric ward. *J Nutr Elder* 1988;**8**:19–30.
32   Cheskin LJ, Kamal N, Crowell MD, Schuster MM, Whitehead WE. Mechanisms of constipation in older persons and effects of fiber compared with placebo. *J Am Geriatr Soc* 1995;**43**:666–9.

33 Hyland CM, Foran JD. Dioctyl sodium sulphosuccinate as a laxative in the elderly. *Practitioner* 1968;**200**:686–9.

34 Wesselius-De Casparis A, Braadbaart S, Bergh-Bohlken GE, Mimica M. Treatment of chronic constipation with lactulose syrup: results of a double-blind study. *Gut* 1968;**9**:84–6.

35 Vanderdonckt J, Coulon J, Denys W, Ravelli GP. Study of the laxative effect of lactitol (importal) in an elderly institutionalised, but not bedridden, population suffering from chronic constipation. *J Clin Exp Gerontol* 1990;**12**: 171–89.

36 Sanders JF. Lactulose syrup assessed in a double-blind study of elderly constipated patients. *J Am Geriatr Soc* 1978;**26**:236–9.

37 Stern FH. Constipation – an omnipresent symptom: effect of a preparation containing prune concentrate and cascarin. *J Am Geriatr Soc* 1966;**14**:1153–5.

38 Marchesi M. A laxative mixture in the therapy of constipation in aged patients. *G Clin Med (Bologna)* 1982;**63**:850–63.

39 Chokhavatia S, Phipps T, Anuras S. Comparative laxation of calcium polycarbophil with psyllium mucilloid in an ambulatory geriatric population. *Curr Ther Res Clin Exp* 1988;**44**:1013–9.

40 Lederle FA, Busch DL, Mattox KM, West MJ, Aske DM. Cost-effective treatment of constipation in the elderly: a randomized double-blind comparison of sorbitol and lactulose. *Am J Med* 1990;**89**:597–601.

41 Doffoel M, Berthel M, Bockel R, Vetter D. Etude comparative du lactitol et du lactulose dans le traitement de la constipation fonctionelle du sujet age. *Med Chir Dig* 1990;**19**:257–9.

42 Williamson J, Coll M, Connolly J. A comparative trial of a new laxative. *Nurs Times* 23 October 1975:1705–7.

43 Fain AM, Susat R, Herring M, Dorton K. Treatment of constipation in geriatric and chronically ill patients: a comparison. *South Med J* 1978;**71**: 677–80.

44 Pers M, Pers B. A crossover comparative study with two bulk laxatives. *J Int Med Res* 1983;**11**:51–3.

45 Kinnunen O, Salokannel J. Constipation in elderly long-stay patients: its treatment by magnesium hydroxide and bulk-laxative. *Ann Clin Res* 1987;**19**: 321–3.

46 Passmore AP, Davies KW, Flanagan PG, Stoker C, Scott MG. A comparison of agiolax and lactulose in elderly patients with chronic constipation. *Pharmacology* 1993;**47**(Suppl 1):249–52.

47 Kinnunen O, Winblad I, Koistenen P, Salokannel J. Safety and efficacy of a bulk laxative containing senna versus lactulose in the treatment of chronic constipation in geriatric patients. *Pharmacology* 1993;**47**(Suppl 1):253–5.

48 Puxty JA, Fox RA. Golytely: a new approach to faecal impaction in old age. *Age Ageing* 1986;**15**:182–4.

49 Kamm MA. Entry criteria for drug trials of irritable bowel syndrome. Review. *Am J Med* 1999;**107**:51S–8S.

50 Tramonte SM, Brand MB, Mulrow CD, Amato MG *et al.* The treatment of chronic constipation in adults. A systematic review. *J Gen Intern Med* 1997;**12**: 15–24.

51 Harari D, Gurwitz JH, Avorn J, Choodnovskiy J, Minaker KL. Correlates of regular laxative use by frail elderly persons. *Am J Med* 1995;**99**:513–8.

52 Glia A, Lindberg G. Quality of life in patients with different types of functional constipation. *Scand J Gastroenterol* 1997;**32**:1083–9.

53 Emmanuel AV, Kamm MA, Roy AJ, Antonelli K. Effect of a novel prokinetic drug, RO93877, on gastrointestinal transit in healthy volunteers. *Gut* 1998;**42**: 511–6.

7 | Access to toilets and toileting

Mandy Fader

Lecturer, Department of Medicine, University College London;
Continence Product Evaluation Network

Research

There is little published research about accessing toilets. Research that has been carried out has mainly focused on the design and utility of commodes and bowel care/shower chairs.

There is some confusion in the literature regarding terminology. Ballinger *et al*[1] have defined the products in the following way:

▪ *Commode:* may be mobile or static. Has a pan (disposable or permanent) and may be used independently of a toilet.

▪ *Sani-chair:* always mobile. Has no pan and is used exclusively over the toilet.

▪ *Shower chair:* always mobile. May be used with or without a pan either in lieu of a toilet or over the toilet.

Nelson *et al*[2] surveyed 147 spinal cord injured patients about their satisfaction and safety with the shower chairs (for bowel care) used in the home. They found that about half the patients were dissatisfied with their chairs and expressed concerns related to:

▪ lack of hand access to perianal area

▪ difficulty in turning and rolling the chair, and

▪ problems with keeping the chair clean.

One-third of the patients experienced chair-related falls, nearly a quarter reported chair-related pressure ulcers and two-thirds of them felt their safety was compromised.

The same group of researchers evaluated three shower chairs using video-taping, photography and questionnaires, and produced performance criteria for the design of an optimal shower chair.[3] Pressure mapping devices were used to measure seat pressures on three subjects who tested all three bowel care/shower chairs to inform seat design.[4] These researchers then designed a more advanced commode-shower chair[5] with lockable, swing-away armrests and lever-activated brakes to facilitate transfers. To prevent pressure ulcers, a chair frame and padding combination was designed to facilitate a seating position that distributed body weight and reduced pressure on pressure points. Cupped, edgeless footrests were designed to reduce the risk of heel ulcers. An adapted version of this chair is now commercially available in the USA.

In the UK, an investigation of commode design by Nazarko[6] highlighted the problem of commodes providing poor trunk support for elderly and disabled people. Prolonged periods of sitting alone (for privacy) to enable defaecation resulted in a risk of falls. Nazarko worked with a manufacturer to produce a design specification for a commode. Consultation with patients indicated that many would prefer to use a toilet. The resulting product was therefore a shower chair which would allow patients to use the product as a commode or which could be wheeled over the toilet.

An evaluation of the four main types of commodes (standard, adjustable height, removable/drop-down arm, adjustable height and removable/drop-down arm combination) was published by the UK Medical Devices Agency in 1993.[7] One-third of the 150 commodes on the market at the time were found to have backwards instability, and most of them scored poorly for aesthetics and comfort. A discussion of the results of this evaluation and its application to nursing was published in 1996.[1]

The maintenance of hospital commodes can be a problem and Gillan[8] complained about the poor condition of commodes in wards for elderly people.

Naylor et al[9] investigated the use of commodes and the attitudes of users and carers towards them in community dwelling patients (115 subjects and 105 carers). The main reasons for commode use were impaired mobility, difficulty climbing stairs and urinary incontinence. Main concerns were lack of privacy and embarrassment about using the commode, unpleasant smells and the poor physical appearance of the commode. Carers tended to view them negatively, particularly with regard to cleaning. Where commodes were used for defaecation in a living area the authors highlighted the problem of odour and recommended the use of a chemical toilet.

Conclusions from research

The conclusions from these studies indicate that improvements in commode design are needed in the following areas:

▪ aesthetics
▪ trunk support
▪ stability (particularly backwards)
▪ adaptability for sideways transfer

- effective brakes for transfer stability
- wheels to provide smooth, easy turning and movement
- pressure ulcer prevention
- foot support
- comfort over long periods
- ease of cleaning.

Informed opinion

Published anecdotal opinion indicates that the practicalities of toileting[10] and bowel management can be difficult for dependent people and that the following factors require attention:

Getting to and onto the toilet, sani-chair/shower chair or commode

- dignity and privacy during transfer (particularly if using a commode/shower chair or hoist)
- safety on transfer to commode/toilet (removable armrests, seats at the same height for lateral transfer, stability of chair/commode)
- appropriate/adapted clothes and underclothes.

Sitting on the toilet, sani-chair/shower chair or commode

- safety and comfort on sitting on the commode/toilet (support from padded armrests and backrests, grab rails to hold on to, toileting sling on hoist)
- provision of optimum position for defaecation (feet on firm surface/platform, slightly raised, leaning slightly forward)
- pressure prevention from hard seating surfaces, for prolonged bowel routines (gel/padded seats)
- ability to summon help (call button/bell).

Maintaining privacy and minimising inhibition during defaecation

- privacy (closed doors/curtains, locks and signs)
- odour control (ventaxia, neutradol, air freshener)
- noise control (noisy ventaxia, radio).

After defaecation

- Bottom wiping (moist toilet tissue, extended bottom wiper, shower unit, portable bidet unit).

Portable receptacles

Bedpans and other portable receptacles are not well described in the literature. Generally, bedpans are considered to be unsuitable for defaecation for safety and acceptability reasons. However, for individuals with specific needs (eg frequency and urgency of defaecation) a portable receptacle may be beneficial. Although many portable urinals are now available for both men and women,[11] very few are recommended for defaecation[12] and they have yet to be formally evaluated.

Summary

Some of these factors (particularly privacy, odour and noise control) are virtually impossible to achieve outside a purpose-built toilet cubicle or room. For this reason *commodes* are likely to be the most *unfavourable* option for toileting and efforts should be focused on making the toilets as accessible as possible to patients, probably by the use of shower chairs.

Exercise, mobility and timing of toileting opportunities

Moderate exercise (cycling or jogging for one hour per day) has been shown to decrease gut transit times significantly and substantially: mean 36 hours compared with 51 hours when 'rest in chair' replaced jogging/ cycling.[13] Although no such study has been carried out in elderly populations, there is some evidence that more frequent toileting (which involves increased mobility) results in more bowel activity. In a trial of prompted voiding for older people in institutional care (primarily for urinary incontinence) Ouslander *et al*[14] found an increase in continent bowel movements, but not a decrease in *incontinent* bowel movements. In terms of timing, it seems likely that toileting after food and/or exercise should make best use of the gastro-colic reflex, although this has not been formally tested in older people.

EVIDENCE-BASED SUMMARY ———————————————————

(*Strength of evidence* [1]–[5]; see Appendix 1)

▪ There are major defects in most of the current designs of shower chairs and commodes including [4]:
  – aesthetics
  – trunk support
  – stability
  – adaptability

- – effective brakes
- – effective wheels
- – pressure ulcer prevention
- – foot support
- – access for cleaning self/user after elimination
- – comfort over long periods
- – ease of cleaning.
- Design specifications for shower chairs that purport to overcome most of the above defects do exist and such chairs have been manufactured, but these 'special' designs are not in common use [4].
- If direct transfer to a toilet is impossible or unsafe, a sani-chair/shower chair is preferable to a commode [4].
- The main concerns of users about commodes are:
  - – lack of privacy
  - – embarrassment over use of commode
  - – unpleasant smells
  - – noise
  - – the poor physical appearance [4].
- Other important considerations of users include:
  - – difficulty with wiping self
  - – stability
  - – difficulty with manoeuvring
  - – ease of cleaning the commode [4].
- The only way to resolve many issues around defaecation is for people to have ready access to toilets and to avoid the use of commodes [5].
- The state of repair of commodes/sani-chairs/shower chairs in institutions is often poor [5].
- Defaecation on a bedpan should be avoided whenever possible [5].
- Increased mobility, exercise and toileting may increase continent bowel activity [4].

WHAT WE DON'T KNOW

- Which commode/sani-chair/shower chair designs (including the special designs) best meet the performance and safety requirements of older people and their carers?
- What sitting position is most effective and acceptable for defaecation and how can it be achieved?

▪ How can toilets be made more accessible, both with and without the use of hoists?

▪ Do strategies to improve privacy improve defaecation?

▪ Which methods of odour and noise control are most acceptable and effective for older people and their carers?

▪ What clothing adaptations/requirements are most acceptable and effective for older people and their carers?

▪ Which methods/tools for bottom wiping are most acceptable and effective for older people and their carers?

▪ What comprises a design specification for a portable receptacle for defaecation?

▪ Are chemical toilets more acceptable for older people and carers in certain community settings?

▪ What toileting products are provided on wards, in residential settings and by home loan stores, and what determines purchasing decisions?

▪ What are the experiences of older people who are toileted using various methods?

Older, dependent people are not a homogeneous group and these questions will need to be applied to different subgroups, for example people living in residential/institutional settings and those living in their own homes.

References

1   Ballinger C, Pain H, Pascoe J, Gore S. Choosing a commode for the ward environment. *Br J Nurs* 1996;**5**:485-6,499–500.

2   Nelson A, Malassigne P, Amerson T, Saltzstein R, Binard J. Descriptive study of bowel care practices and equipment in spinal cord injury. *SCI Nurs* 1993; **10**:65–7.

3   Malassigne P, Nelson A, Amerson T, Salzstein R, Binard J. Toward the design of a new bowel care chair for the spinal cord injured: a pilot study. *SCI Nurs* 1993;**10**:84–90.

4   Nelson AL, Malassigne P, Murray J. Comparison of seat pressures on three bowel care/shower chairs in spinal cord injury. *SCI Nurs* 1994;**11**:105–7.

5   Malassigne P, Nelson AL, Cors MW, Amerson TL. Design of the advanced commode-shower chair for spinal cord-injured individuals. *J Rehabil Res Dev* 1995;**37**:373–82.

6   Nazarko L. Commode design for frail and disabled people. *Prof Nurse* 1995; **11**:95–7.

7   Medical Devices Agency. *Basic Commodes: A Comparative Evaluation.* Disability Equipment Assessment Report A5. London: MDA, October 1993.

8   Gillan J. Seat of the motions. *Nurs Times* 1999;**95**:26.

9   Naylor JR, Mulley GP. Commodes: inconvenient conveniences. *BMJ* 1993; **307**:1258–60.

10   Fader M. Continence. From wheelchairs to toilet. *Nurs Times* 1994;**90**:76–80.

11 Fader M, Pettersson L, Dean G, Brooks R, Cottenden A. The selection of female urinals: results of a multicentre evaluation. *Br J Nurs* 1999;**8**:918–20, 922–5.

12 McIntosh J. Realising the potential of urinals for women. *J Community Nurs* 1998;**12**(8):14–8.

13 Oettle GJ. Effect of moderate exercise on bowel habit. *Gut* 1991;**32**:941–4.

14 Ouslander JG, Simmons S, Schnelle J, Uman G, Fingold S. Effects of prompted voiding on fecal continence among nursing home residents. *J Am Geriatr Soc* 1996;**44**:424–8.

8 | Psychological approaches to bowel care in older people with dementia

Graham Stokes
Consultant Clinical Psychologist, South Staffordshire Healthcare NHS Trust. Lichfield, Staffordshire; Consultant Director of Mental Health, BUPA Care Homes

Behavioural and psychological symptoms of dementia (BPSD) result in treatment with psychotropic medication,

> premature institutionalisation, increased costs of care and significant loss in the quality of life for the patient and his or her family and caregivers.[1]

In the past, these symptoms received less attention than the cognitive changes in dementia. Advances in understanding of the phenomenology, pathobiological, social and environmental origins of BPSD, as well as appreciating that these 'symptoms' are amenable to therapeutic interventions, have promoted active clinical and research interest over the past 15 years. Unfortunately, the challenge of dysfunctional urinary and faecal activity remains largely ignored. A review of the contents of the *International Journal of Geriatric Psychiatry* 1986–2001 yielded just three letters on constipation, urinary incontinence and diarrhoea[2–4] and two papers on behavioural symptoms that referred to faecal smearing[5] and inappropriate urinating.[6] The frequently used assessment instrument for BPSD, the Behavioural Pathology in Alzheimer's Disease Rating Scale (*BEHAVE-AD*)[7] does not record dysfunctional toileting behaviour – yet one of the most difficult and distressing behaviours that carers have to face is when a person with dementia starts to 'wet' or 'soil'.[8] It causes anger and embarrassment, and results in a heavy burden of physical care responsibility.

Toileting difficulty or incontinence

Incontinence, whether urinary or faecal, is rarely an early onset challenge in the major pathologies that cause progressive dementia, namely Alzheimer's disease, vascular dementia and dementia with Lewy bodies. Toileting difficulties are, however, to be expected early in the behavioural profile of dementia.[9]

These apparently contradictory observations are reconciled by asserting that to be found wet or soiled does not automatically provide evidence of incontinence. Incontinence denotes a failure of the controls associated with normal bladder and bowel function. It is therefore an *explanation* for impaired toileting performance, not a *description* of that activity. A toileting difficulty may also arise when bowel function is unimpaired because the achievement and maintenance of continence is a complex skill involving many cortical, psychological, physical, sensory and environmental factors. Hence, while the person may possess bowel control, this may not result in the acceptable passing of faeces.

The practice of assessment

The label to be employed advisedly when a person soils themselves is 'toileting difficulty', which leads logically to the question 'why?'. Before examining the possible explanations, behavioural labels are, at best, the first step on the assessment path.

Behavioural labels

Stokes[9] developed a tripartite structure of assessment for challenging behaviour in dementia. This commences with the label, but then progresses to the formulation of an 'operational definition', a description rich in accurate detail and composed of two elements:

1 *Behavioural definition:* a precise description of the essential details and parameters of dysfunctional behaviour revealing the observable nature of the problem. Once the behaviour is defined, the 'label' can be used judiciously as all on the care/clinical team know what is meant by the term and its use will be challenged if it is employed otherwise.

2 *Behavioural characteristics:* a description of 'what the behaviour looks like'; in other words, what the person actually does. In practice, a person's behaviour would be described in terms unique to them and their circumstances: a process known as *pinpointing*.[10] Ethological research over the past 15 years has, however, yielded broad descriptive categories of many challenging behaviours in dementia, including the problems of toileting.[9–12]

The behavioural definition together with the behavioural characteristics comprise the operational definition that precisely details the behaviour in question. This enables us to move on from understanding the nature of the action to an appreciation of explanation. Explanations that are rich and varied may have little to do with neuropathology, for when:

we follow any person's dementing illness carefully, observing its course in the realities of everyday life, it is extremely difficult to conclude that we are simply witnessing the inexorable consequences of a process of degeneration in nervous tissue.[13]

This understanding has enabled the development of a person-centred model of understanding that addresses the subjective experience of dementia.[14,15] It is a model that does not deny the contribution of neuropathology, but which also reveals a person who is unique, yet one with whom we have so much in common, an individual struggling to survive and communicate behind a barrier of intellectual and linguistic destruction.

Box 1 demonstrates how the tripartite model of assessment is applied to the impairment of toileting skills. The behavioural definition does not discriminate on the basis of presumed intent but focuses on the deficient toileting actions. The behavioural characteristics have been established during observational research as the most commonly occurring actions. Some are passive, others active; some people are discreet, the behaviour

Box 1. Application of a tripartite structure of assessment to the impairment of toileting skills

Label		Toileting difficulty
	O	
	P	
Behavioural definition	E	The voiding of urine or faeces following either
	R	an unsuccessful effort, or with no apparent
	A	attempt to employ an acceptable facility
	T	(eg toilet, commode, urine bottle)
	I	
Behavioural characteristics	O	Parcelling (eg wrapping and concealing the
	N	evidence in drawers, cupboards, etc)
	A	
	L	Wetting or soiling clothes:
		– while sitting (passive)
	D	– while standing or walking (active)
	E	
	F	Wetting or soiling the bed (passive)
	I	
	N	Using an inappropriate receptacle
	I	(eg bin, fire bucket)
	T	
	I	Urinating against wall
	O	
	N	Smearing

of others is invasive. Pinpointing the nature of their conduct provides clues as to why it may be occurring, for example:

■ parcelling: spite, embarrassment
■ passive soiling: incontinence, depression, fear
■ smearing: curiosity
■ active soiling: apraxia, disorientation, poor mobility
■ inappropriate receptacle: agnosia.

Seeking an explanation

To understand the complexity of causation is to appreciate that toileting is the result of negotiating an intricate chain of behaviour that commences with the recognition of need and concludes with the successful passing of faeces (Box 2). In reality, the elements of the chain are not separate and independent atoms of behaviour but interrelated skills and actions. The chain of behaviour can break down at any point because of disease, disability, emotional disorder, environmental factors or a mixture of all these. Disturbance of the skills chain results in dysfunctional bowel movement.

Potential explanations

Rich data have been obtained on the possible reasons for dysfunctional toileting actions by watching the actions of carers, talking to both

---

Box 2. The essential pathway to successful toileting

1 Recognising the need, and postponing within limits, the act of passing urine and faeces (failure = incontinence)
2 Being motivated to use the toilet
3 Possessing the physical strength and steadiness to stand
4 Possessing the mobility and confidence to cover the distance to the toilet and overcome any obstacles on the way (eg floor coverings, stairs, outstretched legs of others)
5 Maintaining goal-oriented behaviour
6 Being able to locate the toilet (or acceptable alternative)
7 Perceiving and experiencing the toilet as accessible, safe, hygienic and private
8 Possessing the dexterity and co-ordination to adjust clothing
9 Initiating the act

caregivers and those who need to be cared for, whether at home, in day care or residential and hospital settings, and also by observation of those with dementia.

Faecal incontinence

Failure or impairment of bowel control may cause involuntary soiling. Such dysfunction may arise as a result of bowel problems, diabetes mellitus or cortical atrophy.

Inappropriate bowel activity

An awareness of need which does not result in acceptable toileting behaviour may lead to inappropriate bowel activity. There are several common explanations.

Neuropsychological dysfunction

- *Expressive aphasia* will interfere with a person's capacity to communicate the need to pass faeces. Thus, a request for assistance to stand or locate the toilet may flounder on the rock of their disintegrated 'dementia speech'. Hence, their need will remain unacknowledged.
- *Receptive aphasia* will mean that requests to toilet or a query as to whether a person requires assistance may not be understood.
- *Visual agnosia* is a disorder of recognition that results in an inability to identify an object, such as a toilet, by vision alone. Similar objects, such as a washbasin or bath, may be used instead.
- *Spatial agnosia*, a variation of visual agnosia, is an inability to find one's way around even familiar places. It looks like disorientation, but is not produced by memory impairment.
- *Unilateral visual inattention or one-side neglect* results in a person not 'seeing' anything, normally to their left.[16] As a result, they bump into things and fail to see objects. The implications for toileting are easy to appreciate.
- *Apraxias* interfere with toileting performance:
  - *ideational apraxia*: a complex task involving a series of movements cannot be performed. Order and sequencing are lost once the action is under voluntary control and the task becomes 'completely disordered'.[16]
  - *dressing apraxia*: attempts to dress result in disorganised actions as the person fails to relate clothing appropriately to their body. A consequence is the inability to achieve the appropriate arrangement of clothing prior to toileting. The result is soiled clothing.

Disorientation

Toileting difficulties can arise following a move to new surroundings. Some-one unfamiliar with their environment may roam around the building searching for the toilet until they are compelled to soil themselves. It does not matter how often they are told, they will never learn, for the inability to store information works against the acquisition of information. Even when a person has lived for many years in the same house they will eventually become disoriented as their recall of once familiar places and layout is affected by the progressive loss of stored memories.

Environment

Even when a person with dementia is aware of the location of the toilet, the design and layout of the building may make reaching it difficult. The outcome of the 'race' between bowel and legs may depend on the distance which has to be covered and the strength and confidence the person possesses to avoid obstacles which may bar the way. Some obstacles may be obvious (eg stairs, steps and heavy doors) and others may not (eg non-slip shiny floors that look wet and slippery to a pair of aged eyes, or a pattern on the floor or carpet that may suggest a step).

Loss of goal-directed behaviour

A person with dementia may get out of their chair with the objective of using the toilet, but then forget what they had intended to do. The frag-mentation of experience may leave them walking apparently aimlessly with no obvious motive, until the urge is so great that they soil themselves wherever they may be.

Mobility and dexterity

Toileting difficulties may be the indirect consequence of physical disability. Despite being able to recognise the need to use the toilet, a person with dementia may be prevented from doing so because of unsteadiness while walking or standing or because of slowness in moving. Alternatively, the person may reach the toilet in time, but have problems opening the door or adjusting their clothing because fine hand movements are compromised by the effects of arthritis or tremor associated with Parkinson's disease.

Depression

The appearance of a toileting difficulty may be the result of clinical depression. Older people with dementia are far (perhaps ten times) more likely to suffer from depression than those who are not. Contrary to belief, loss of insight offers no protection. It is now widely accepted that depression in dementia demands vigorous treatment.[17] Loss of interest, poor concentration, apathy and withdrawal combine to interfere seriously with toileting performance.

Apathy

Continence is an acquired habit, the motivation for which may diminish in old age with loss of strength and stamina. As life becomes effortful, older adults conserve energy; for a minority of those with dementia this may result in a disinclination to toilet appropriately.

Fear

A person with dementia may be frightened of falling, entering the unknown, negotiating stairs or becoming lost. If people feel frightened, that is what matters – whether or not we assess them as competent. Fear comes from within and is often impervious to the reassuring words of others. Fear may be exaggerated by sensory impairment or generated by perceptual distortions.

Embarrassment

Exposed to degrading care procedures, being too embarrassed to ask or fearful of humiliation if they were to soil themselves on the way to the toilet may result in a person discreetly passing faeces. Unfortunately, attempts to preserve dignity may result in condemnation and inevitable embarrassment. In advanced dementia, embarrassment after having soiled may result in parcelling.

Curiosity

Curiosity is an explanation especially pertinent at times of abnormal bowel movements (eg constipation and diarrhoea) and may account for faecal smearing. Curiosity impels much of what we do. Berlyne coined the term 'epistemic behaviour' or 'knowledge augmenting behaviour'.[18] It is suggested that not knowing sets up a state of emotional tension which is diminished by seeking knowledge. To acquire knowledge, the environment is explored.

When cognitive destruction is advanced and a person no longer understands their own bodily functions, behaviour may degenerate to a state that others see as degrading. Few who smear faeces do so to be maliciously destructive; most are simply correcting the consequences of their own curiosity. A person with dementia who is slowed by age, whose dexterity is affected by arthritis and whose co-ordination of clothing is damaged by dressing apraxia may unknowingly be sitting on a toilet with their clothes rucked up beneath them. As they open their bowels, their disordered bowel movement compounds their discomfort and, with impaired judgement and impoverished reasoning, they commit an act they would never have previously done. To investigate why they feel so uncomfortable they place their hands within their clothing and, on removal, find them covered in faeces. Attempts to remove it by wiping or shaking it off then occur. Within a short passage of time, the fading of the memory trace typical of the storage deficits observed in Alzheimer's disease results in the fragmentation of experience. The act has not been committed. However, they still feel uncomfortable and – as if for the first time, and to them the subjective reality is that it is – they place their hands behind them. Each investigation and subsequent attempt to remove the faeces result in what we see as smearing.

Self-determination

The desire to exercise agency in intimate self-care may be so strong as to result in valiant, albeit unsuccessful, attempts to demonstrate independence or a refusal either to ask for, or to accept, assistance.

Manipulation, attention seeking and spite

The purpose of inappropriate toileting is to exercise a negative effect on another person. The motivation is to get one's own way, attract attention or retaliate. As cognitive capacity is required to set such objectives, this explanation is valid only at the beginnings of dementia and invariably provides evidence of dysfunctional relationships.

Inadequate facilities

In communal arrangements (eg day centres, residential homes or hospital wards) the number of toilets available may be inadequate to meet the needs of those required to use them. This is especially pertinent at times of peak demand, for example following meal times. The toilets may be difficult to enter, unclean or smell of stale urine, poorly lit, too public or lack adaptations to make them safe. On their own, these failings do not result in inappropriate toileting, but they discourage use and, as a result, may create delay as the person embarks upon a potentially fruitless search for an acceptable toilet. The outcome is episodes of soiling.

Over-dependency

Over-concern by a family carer or the de-skilling effects of 'disempowerment' and institutionalisation may lead to the premature loss of independent will and a regression to 'infantile' dependency.

Drug effects

Toileting difficulties may be a sign of drug side effects. For example, they may be attributable to excessive drowsiness caused by tranquillisers, or soiling at night may arise following the prescription of night-time sedation. Nasman *et al*[5] associated faecal smearing with the use of benzodiazepines.

Summary of potential explanations for dysfunctional toileting

Toileting difficulties are by no means straightforward problems to understand. Motivation and action are also enshrined within a person's biography and influenced by personal habit. The range of explanation is also affected by the progression of the presumptive disease. For example, motivational factors are in part dependent on cognitive competence. Does the person possess insight? To what extent can experience be retained and recalled, and reason exercised?

Identification of cause may also by hindered by the hidden nature of the behaviour. It can be difficult to identify accurately an incident of 'soiling' at the time of its occurrence if, for example, the person is either discreet, indifferent or unaware of their bodily functions. There is no simple solution to this difficulty.

Finally – this applies to all conduct that is challenging – a person's behaviour is not only unique to them but the same behavioural phenotype can occur at different times for different reasons. To gain a genuine understanding of a person's behaviour it needs to be understood as it is occurring *now*. The case of Wendy, a woman with dementia, illustrates how the reasons for a previous episode of toileting difficulty may have little bearing on the explanation for this or the next challenging incident.[10]

Case example: The trials of Wendy, aged 47 years, a woman with chronic-progressive multiple sclerosis and dementia

Wendy's husband could cope with much, but her wetting and soiling was beyond the pale. He would regularly ask whether she needed the toilet, invariably to be told 'no' or to be met with silence. Then some time later she would be found with clothes soiled or there would be urine and faeces in the bed or on the toilet floor. Her rejection of his help angered him, yet what really infuriated him was that her toileting difficulties were less severe at the day centre. Her actions at home seemed deliberate. One day, having found his wife soiled on the way to the lavatory, just moments after asking her whether she needed the toilet, he flew into a rage and grabbed hold of her. The casualty officer's report documented two broken fingers and a dislocated thumb.

There was no single reason for Wendy's behaviour, but several reasons, some of which she found impossible to articulate:

■ *Damaged sphincter control:* incontinence is a common feature of multiple sclerosis (MS), and at times Wendy failed to acknowledge her need to toilet.

■ *Fatigue:* The tiredness and loss of stamina experienced by people with MS significantly interfere with efficiency in daily life. Wendy would spend much of her time lying on the bed, too tired to respond to her responsibilities and needs.

■ *Physical limitations on movement:* Wendy had lost her sight in one eye and suffered from weakness and spasticity on her right side. As a result, her movements were slow and her co-ordination poor.

■ *Exaggerated forgetfulness:* Wendy's dementia was mild, yet sufficient to compromise her memory and concentration. When somewhere new, she would sometimes struggle to locate the toilet even when reminded.

■ *Depression:* the most frequently observed emotional disturbance in MS is low mood. Wendy's family doctor had been treating her for depression for nearly two years, with little success.

■ *Forlorn attempts to maintain independence:* Wendy is proud. She is determined to maintain her self-respect, even though her physical weakness renders her increasingly dependent and likely to fail.

■ *Spite:* marital tensions pre-existed Wendy's MS. Her husband continued to live his life, often leaving her alone in the evening and she would retaliate by soiling when he was out. This also enabled her to exercise a degree of control over her husband's activity.

■ *Embarrassment:* in the absence of love and tenderness, she found personal care at the hands of her husband awkward and embarrassing. She would rather try herself than experience the indignity of revealing her intimate needs to him.

Functional analysis

The pursuit of understanding has been advanced by a move away from unstructured and intuitive theorising to systematic and direct observation of behaviour, with the objective of establishing whether there is a relationship between the action and its context.

Behavioural analysis, often referred to as an ABC analysis, establishes over a defined period the antecedents (A) and consequences (C) of a defined behaviour (B) in order to establish which aspects of a person's environment serve to trigger or maintain the dysfunctional act. However, from what is known about dementia, at least in cases of advanced dementia recall deficits invariably militate against the maintenance of behaviour by a learned appreciation of the consequences that will follow.

Behavioural analysis provides a detailed description of the relationship between environmental events and behaviour, but it is a limited methodology. Certainly, incidents of inappropriate bowel movements occur in a particular setting and may be inextricably related to that situation and its broader context but, as revealed in the taxonomy of possible explanations, actions are also a function of the person and their motivations. Functional analysis builds on the empirical rigour of behavioural analysis and addresses the function served by the behaviour. Moniz-Cook *et al*[19] employed functional analysis to understand the fear felt by a woman who refused to use the toilet.

Researchers have identified 'the functional significance of even the most bizarre and serious behaviours'.[20] Functional analysis does not restrict itself to an appreciation of the immediate antecedents and/or consequences of a behaviour, but attempts to gain an understanding of the meaning and function of a particular behaviour, in a particular set of circumstances, for a particular individual.[20]

Intervention

Contemporary psychological interventions are founded on the insights provided by robust observational methods and functional analysis. The objective is to resolve rather than manage inappropriate bowel activity.

Multimodal intervention is a preventive methodology that constitutes a global environmental response to the challenge of dependency that trawls the known causes of toileting difficulties and attempts to avoid, compensate for or accommodate the reasons for a person with dementia being found wet or soiled.[10] Goal planning is a structured approach that draws upon a person's remaining strengths in order to help and motivate them towards tackling their difficulties and meeting their needs.[21] For those who are incontinent or no longer motivated to use the toilet, interventions are limited in ambition and take the form of an individualised approach to habit retraining. This uses a person's pattern of bowel activity to guide a toileting programme of checks and prompts.[10]

Despite the increasing application of psychological methods, there are only isolated examples of single-case experimental studies to validate the utility of these methods.[6,19] Anecdotal evidence and clinical case-work have provided evidence of therapeutic achievement over the past decade. The paucity of methodologically sound clinical trials in BPSD is well acknowledged[22] and has led many to argue that therapeutic interventions have yet to become evidence-based.[23] It certainly cannot be said that such interventions constitute the nursing care norm. Most nurses and social care staff receive no training in – and are thus unaware of – psychological and behavioural principles, so that the potential for resolution is not appreciated. The management of bowel problems therefore continues unchanged, invariably founded on scheduled toileting and controlled evacuation.

EVIDENCE-BASED SUMMARY

(*Strength of evidence* [1]–[5]; see Appendix 1)

▪ Toileting difficulties occur early in the behavioural profile of dementia [2].

▪ Observational research identifies recurring behavioural characteristics in demented subjects which provide a challenge to the management of bowel function [4].

▪ Multiple neurological and psychological changes associated with the dementing process contribute to abnormal behaviour in bowel management [4].

▪ Multimodal intervention with goal setting can enable bowel problems to be avoided, compensated for or accommodated [4].

WHAT WE DON'T KNOW

▪ The absence of clinical research evidence reflects therapeutic nihilism in the domain of bowel management within dementia care. This needs to be addressed if psychological interventions are to be evidence-based.

▪ Would improvements in the skills base of nursing and dementia care staff improve competence in observation, analysis and psychological interventions?

▪ Would improved availability of formal specialist support to nursing homes overcome the 'isolation of care' in these environments?[24]

▪ What should be the funding arrangements and pathways of 'outreach' healthcare support to ensure appropriate levels of expert bowel care for a patient constituency unable to articulate their health needs?

References

1   Finkel SI, Costa E, Silva J, Cohen G, Miller S, Sartorius N. Behavioral and psychological signs and symptoms of dementia: a consensus statement on current knowledge and implications for research and treatment. Review. *Int Psychogeriatr* 1996;8(Suppl 3):497–500.

2   MacDonald AJ. Protocols for constipation and urinary incontinence. *Int J Geriatr Psychiatry* 1993;**8**:269.

3   Flint AJ, Skelly JM. The management of urinary incontinence in dementia. *Int J Geriatr Psychiatry* 1994;**9**:245.

4   Shah A. Infective diarrhoea on hospital-based psychogeriatric wards. *Int J Geriatr Psychiatry* 1994;**9**:74.

5   Nasman B, Bucht G, Eriksson S, Sandman PO. Behavioural symptoms in the institutional elderly – relationship to dementia. *Int J Geriatr Psychiatry* 1993; **8**:843–9.

6   Bird M, Alexopoulos P, Adamowicz J. Success and failure in five case studies: use of cued recall to ameliorate behaviour problems in senile dementia. *Int J Geriatr Psychiatry* 1995;**10**:305–11.

7   Reisberg B, Borenstein J, Salob SP, Ferris SH *et al.* Behavioral symptoms in Alzheimer's disease: phenomenology and treatment. *J Clin Psychiatry* 1987; **48**(Suppl):9–15.

8   Gilleard CJ. *Living with Dementia.* London: Croom Helm, 1984.

9   Stokes G. Incontinent or not? Don't label: describe and assess. *J Dem Care* 1995;**3**(1):20–1.

10 Stokes G. *Challenging Behaviour in Dementia: a Person-centred Approach.* Bicester: Winslow Press, 2000.

11 Stokes G. *Common Problems with the Elderly Confused: Incontinence and Inappropriate Urinating.* Bicester: Winslow Press, 1987.

12 Stokes G. In: Stokes G, Goudie F (eds). The management of toileting difficulties. *Working with Dementia.* Bicester, Winslow Press, 1990.

13 Kitwood T. In: Woods RT (ed). A dialectical framework for dementia. *Handbook of the Clinical Psychology of Ageing.* Chichester: John Wiley, 1996.

14 Kitwood T. Person and process in dementia. *Int J Geriatr Psychiatry* 1993;**9**: 541–5.

15 Stokes G. In: Woods RT (ed). Challenging behaviour in dementia: a psychological approach. *Handbook of the Clinical Psychology of Ageing.* Chichester: John Wiley, 1996.

16 Holden UP. *Ageing, Neuropsychology and the 'New Dementias'.* London: Chapman & Hall, 1995.

17 Baldwin RC. In: Jacoby R, Oppenheimer C (eds). Depressive illness. *Psychiatry in the Elderly,* 2nd edn. Oxford: Oxford University Press, 1997.

18 Berlyne DE. *Conflict, Arousal and Curiosity.* New York: McGraw-Hill, 1960.

19 Moniz-Cook E, Stokes G, Agar S. Difficult behaviour and dementia in nursing homes: five cases of psychosocial intervention. *Int J Clin Psychol Psychother* (in press).

20 Samson DM, McDonnell AA. Functional analysis and challenging behaviours. *Behav Psycho* 1990;**18**:259–72.

21 Barrowclough C, Fleming I. *Goal Planning with Elderly People.* Manchester: Manchester University Press, 1986.

22 Finkel S. Introduction to behavioural and psychological symptoms of dementia (BPSD). *Int J Geriatr Psychiatry* 2000;**15**(Suppl 1):S2–S4.

23 Bleathman C, Morton I. In: Burns A, Levy R (eds). Psychological Treatments. *Dementia.* London: Chapman & Hall Medical, 1994.

24 Jackson GA, Templeton GJ, Whyte J. An overview of behaviour difficulties found in long-term elderly care settings. *Int J Geriatr Psychiatry* 1999;**14**:426–30.

9 | The older person's viewpoint: feedback from interviews with older people

Background

The involvement of older people and carers in the formulation of standards is not only essential but is now a core feature of national plans to improve the quality of care.[1]

The inclusion of older people suffering with bowel problems within the workshop was considered and discussed with representatives of patient/carer organisations. It was felt that such a meeting would be potentially challenging for older people and a difficult environment in which to discuss such personal issues. It was therefore planned to feed back the deliberations of the working group to older people with bowel problems to determine whether there were issues of concern that had been ignored and to establish the priorities for the management of bowel care as perceived by older people.

The following feedback is derived from interviews conducted by *In*contact* with people suffering from bowel problems.

Specific issues

A number of aspects of management were felt to be particularly important.

Patient dignity/nursing care

The following issues were highlighted:

- use of toilet as opposed to commode whenever possible
- clean working facilities
- the need to accept that people with faecal incontinence will have accidents and should not be blamed
- timely response to call/bell for assistance
- fluid intake, eating meals and mobility need encouragement and monitoring
- compliance with medication should be monitored
- healthcare assistants should not be left without supervision by qualified nursing staff.

---

*In*contact, United House, North Road, London N7 9DP.

Access to care

A specialist continence advisory service should be available to all older people. The perceived view from older people is that many of them are not being offered this support. Services for urinary incontinence may be available but those for faecal incontinence are often not available.

All older people requiring acute or longer-term care should receive a full bowel function assessment by a trained practitioner. Where the assessment shows the need, a referral to a continence nurse specialist or other relevant medical specialty should be made.

Older people should have access to appropriate means of managing their bowel problems, including incontinence pads. Pads need to be provided in sufficient quantity and quality to be changed at regular intervals during the day.

Toilets and toileting

Commodes should be used only when a trip to the toilet is not possible. They should not be used to save time in taking someone to the toilet.

Commodes and toilets should be kept scrupulously clean and regularly checked for cleanliness and damage. Where possible, outdated commodes should be replaced with newer commodes.

Methods for facilitating bottom wiping need to be given due attention. Training for staff and older people may be required to ensure the best possible care. Toilet paper should be within reach – the back of the commode is not within reach for many people.

Fluid intake

The importance of access to fluid needs to be stressed. Water should be available in glasses within easy reach, as well as assistance to help very frail older people to drink. Guidance on fluid intake would be appreciated by older people, ie how much fluid is appropriate.

Care pathways/professional education

Older people perceive that often the attitude is that nothing can be done about faecal incontinence and that it is the individual's own fault. The individual and health workers may wish to avoid the issue and to ignore or deny that the problem exists. It is also perceived that sometimes services, support and advice are not available unless someone 'kicks up a fuss'.

For these reasons, educational programmes are needed for health workers. Some type of standardised care pathway for the management of bowel problems would be a helpful outcome from the workshop.

Information

Older people should be provided with information about their bowel condition and given explanations of possible treatment and management options. Such information should be backed up with written information with large print available.

An example was given of an older person who felt that more information should have been provided, as well as discussion about the possible advantages of a colostomy and further information on dietary modification and odour control.

Older people with bowel problems should have access to support groups such as *In*contact.

Reference

1   Department of Health. *Essence of Care: Patient-focused Benchmarking for Health Care Practitioners*. London: DH, 2001.

10 | A professional's perspective: how to change practice

Linda Nazarko

Director, Nightingale Nursing Home, London;
Visiting Senior Lecturer, South Bank University

Introduction

Constipation is perceived to be common in older people, but evidence suggests that ageing does not lead to constipation and that a healthy 85 year old is no more likely to be constipated than a healthy 20 year old.[1] However, both constipation and laxative use are highest in older adults, with 79% of those in hospitals, 59% in nursing homes and 38% living at home regularly prescribed laxatives.[2] Millions of pounds are spent each year on laxative prescriptions.

Research on the prevalence of bowel dysfunction in older people living in nursing homes is scant. Research in the USA indicates that 12.5% of older people admitted to nursing homes suffer from constipation, and a further 7% develop constipation within three months of entering a nursing home.[3] The average nursing home resident is 85 years old. It has also been found that people aged 95 or over are more likely to suffer from constipation than those below 95.[4]

There is little research on the costs of prescribing for nursing home residents. The costs of prescribing laxatives are generally 'lost' within the budgets of general practitioners (GPs) who provide medical care for nursing home residents. Nursing homes do not collate such data because the costs of laxatives, enemas and suppositories are met from NHS budgets and not immediately evident to nurse managers. One study which matched nursing home residents and older people living at home found that the mean prescribing cost for a nursing home resident was £45.27 per month – three times the cost of prescribing for people of a similar age living at home. Factors leading to increased costs were much higher levels of laxative and anti-ulcer medication. The average nursing home resident was prescribed 5.6 medications per day, while the average older person living at home was prescribed 2.6 medications per day.[5]

There is little literature on assessment and management of constipation within nursing homes.[6,7] Studies that have been published concentrate on medication to treat constipation.[8,9]

Review of available evidence

The available evidence suggests that ageing is not synonymous with an increased incidence of constipation, but that older people living in nursing homes are more likely to be prescribed more medications than those living at home. Many medications commonly prescribed to nursing home residents can increase the risk of constipation.

Nursing home residents are more frail than older people living at home. Immobility is a major problem, with 78% of people admitted to nursing homes unable to transfer from bed to chair unaided. Many nursing home residents have neurological diseases such as Parkinson's disease and stroke that make mobility difficult and predispose to constipation.

Informed opinion

My informed opinion is based on my research and experience. I have managed nursing homes since 1986. In 1996, I surveyed the educational needs of nursing home nurses. In 1996 and 1997 I researched rehabilitation and quality of care in UK nursing homes for my MSc dissertation, surveying 1,000 beds in South Thames and conducting action research in three homes over a period of 12 weeks. This research involved working with the nursing staff and verifying the data collected on the survey. In 1998, I was appointed Director of Nursing for the Registered Nursing Home Association (RNHA) and over two years worked closely with 1,500 homes that were members of RNHA. I then returned to managing a home, Nightingale Nursing Home.

Current practice

Constipation and bowel disorders experienced by frail older people are poorly managed in the NHS, independent and voluntary sectors. When an older person complains of constipation, the usual response is to prescribe laxatives. Constipation is viewed as a disease and the 'pill for every ill' mentality swings into play. Each time a laxative is prescribed without investigating the cause of the constipation a health promotion opportunity is lost and the cycle of laxative misuse perpetuated. In my experience, bowel care receives less attention than it did 15 years ago, both in hospitals and nursing homes. Routine monitoring of bowel actions is considered to be outmoded. Now that the bowel book or chart is no longer used to monitor bowel actions it is not uncommon for people to be discharged from hospital faecally impacted. Nurses working in hospitals also report cases where older people admitted from nursing homes with acute abdominal pain are found to be faecally impacted. Nursing staff seem to rely more on aperients, and use enemas and suppositories less frequently. This is not always appropriate.

Barriers to change

Nurses face a heavy workload. Nursing home residents and hospital patients are more dependent and more likely to develop bowel problems than people who are well. The nursing workforce is less stable. The national shortage of registered nurses has led to increased reliance on agency and bank staff. These nurses rarely work for a long period on the same unit, which affects their ability to work as efficiently and effectively as regular staff. Full-time staff are under increased strain and pressure. In this situation, time horizons shrink to getting through the shift and staff seldom consider proactive work.

The time nurses spend in face-to-face contact with patients has fallen as demands for increased record keeping have grown. In recent years tasks such as taking blood and changing suprapubic catheters, once considered a doctor's role, have been taken over by nurses. In the face of these pressures, nurses have given less priority to traditional roles. The body responsible for registering and regulating nurses prior to the intro-duction of the Nursing and Midwifery Council recently felt it necessary to emphasise that serving meals and feeding patients were a nurse's role.

Most nursing homes care for older people. Older adults living in nursing homes have complex needs, yet only a small number of nurses caring for older people have any qualifications in gerontology.[10] National minimum standards introduced in 2002 specify the size of rooms and width of doorways – but do not require nurses to have specialist qualifica-tions in the care of older people.[11] The perception is that anyone can nurse older people and that no specialist skills are required.[12]

It is difficult for nurses who do not have a good knowledge base to offer holistic care to a vulnerable group.[13] Lack of knowledge of gerontology and the physiology of the bowel means that nurses may be unaware of what can be done to resolve problems in frail older people, so there is little impetus for change.

Practical experiences of change management

While manager of the nursing home, I introduced a bowel management programme[14] as part of a long-term programme to improve quality of care. Our first attempt to improve bowel care was unsuccessful and was abandoned, leaving the nurses with a feeling of failure.

Box 1. Components of bowel management programme

▪ Enhance resident mobility
▪ Ensure residents have sufficient fluids
▪ Review medications that could cause bowel disease
▪ Provide a diet high in fibre
▪ Ensure residents have privacy and time to open bowels
▪ Encourage residents to use the toilet after breakfast
▪ Ensure availability of suitable toilet adaptations and alternatives to suit individual needs
▪ Monitor bowel actions
▪ Carry out bowel assessments

Six months later we discussed why bowel management had not improved, and found that it was because a simplistic approach had been adopted to bowel care – adding bran to diets, and expecting that all problems would be solved. It was decided to spend three months working and planning before making another attempt to improve bowel care. We examined the research, looked at our practice and at the factors that would contribute to change, involving both medical colleagues and our chefs. Box 1 outlines the changes that were made.

Nurses were not resistant to change[15] – they wanted to improve the quality of care – but the greatest barrier to change was the fear of failure. I had to work hard to assure staff that even though not every change was successful, change provided the opportunity to learn and ultimately to improve practice. The nursing staff also worried about the medical staff's attitude to their work. In fact, the doctors were supportive and helped enormously both by saying that they felt that bowel care was really the province of the nurse and also by changing, discontinuing and reviewing medication such as codeine-based analgesics that were contributing to constipation. They were also at hand if any abnormalities were discovered when bowel assessments were carried out, such as anal fissure, haemorrhoids or (on one occasion) a carcinoma.

Subtle modifications were made by the chefs to the diet provided, such as adding beans and pulses to casseroles and using a mixture of wholemeal and white flour in cakes and puddings.

Some problems in general application of the bowel programme

This bowel programme has now been used by many other homes in the UK, but some matron managers have reported problems in the following areas.

General practitioners

In some larger homes several GPs are involved whereas in our nursing home there were only two. It is more difficult to work with medical staff in a large home where several GPs are involved. Some large homes solved this problem by developing a structure in which a doctor is responsible for a group of patients on one unit or floor. This enables medical and nursing staff to work together and offer less fragmented care.

Menu planning

Some larger homes and groups of homes have central menu planning which managers find difficult to influence. This makes it difficult to increase the amount of fibre offered to residents. In one home, a manager eventually overcame this by using juiced fruits to increase the fibre content of diets.

WHAT WE DON'T KNOW

The following issues require further exploration:

▪ What is the most effective method (including non-laxative methods) for promoting normal bowel actions in frail older people?

▪ Does a nurse-led bowel management programme improve outcomes for faecal incontinence and constipation?

▪ What is the role of therapy assessment for facilitating toileting in nursing homes?

▪ What is the cost-effectiveness of different management regimens?

▪ How can medical and nursing staff best be educated to ensure that bowel dysfunction is investigated and treated?

▪ What is the best design for toilets to enable frail people to retain privacy and dignity when defaecating?

▪ How can toilet seats be modified to prevent discomfort?

▪ Is there evidence that fluid/fibre/caffeine/artificial sweeteners promote improved bowel care?

References

1   Heaton KW, Radvan H, Cripps H, Mountford RA *et al.* Defaecation frequency and timing, and stool form in the general population: a prospective study. *Gut* 1992;**33**:818–24.

2   Kinnunen O. Study of constipation in a geriatric hospital, day hospital, old people's home and at home. *Aging (Milano)* 1991;**3**:161–70.

3   Robson KM, Kiely DK, Lembo T. Development of constipation in nursing home residents. *Dis Colon Rectum* 2000;**43**:940–3.

4   Fries BE, Morris JN, Skarupski KA, Blaum CS *et al.* Accelerated dysfunction among the very oldest-old in nursing homes. *J Gerontol A Biol Sci Med Sci* 2000;**55**:M336–41.

5   Avery AJ, Groom LM, Brown KP, Thornhill K, Boot D. The impact of nursing home patients on prescribing costs in general practice. *J Clin Pharm Ther* 1999;**24**:357–63.

6   Nazarko L. Elderly care counts. Power to the people. *Nurs Times* 1996;**92**: 48–9.

7   Nazarko L. Commode design for frail and disabled people. *Prof Nurse* 1995; **11**:2:95–7.

8   Ungar A. Movicol in treatment of constipation and faecal impaction. *Hospital Med* 2000;**61**:37–40.

9   Thacker E. *Movicol in the management of constipation in patients with neurological diseases: an open study in nursing home residents.* Presented at the 21st Annual Conference and Exhibition of the Association for Continence Advice, Torquay, 21–24th May, 2001.

10 Nazarko L. The educational needs of nursing home nurses. *Nurs Times – Learning Curve* 1998; **2**(7):2–3.

11 Department of Health. *National minimum standards for care homes for older people.* London: DH, 2001.

12 Nazarko L. Heading back to the workhouse. *Elder care* 1998;**10**:8–10.

13 Nazarko L. Nursing home nurses need support to update skills. *Nurs Times* 1996;**92**:38–40.

14 Nazarko L. Preventing constipation in older people. Review. *Prof Nurse* 1996; **11**:816–8.

15 East L, Robinson J. Change in process: bringing about change in health care through action research. *J Clin Nurs* 1994;**3**:57–61.

Appendix 1

Grading used for strength of evidence and recommendations

The grading below is used by the International Consultation on Urological Diseases (ICUD) and is based on the recommendations of the Oxford Centre for Evidence-Based Medicine.[1]

LEVELS OF EVIDENCE

Level 1   Includes one or more randomised controlled trials (RCTs) or 'all or none' studies in which no treatment is not an option.

Level 2   Includes good quality prospective 'cohort studies'. These may include a single group when individuals who develop the condition are matched from within the original cohort group. There can be parallel cohorts where those with the condition in the first group are matched by those in the second group.

Level 3   Includes good quality retrospective 'case-control studies' where a group of patients who have a condition are matched (for sex, age etc) by control individuals from a general population.

Level 4   Includes good quality 'case series' where a group of patients, all with the same condition/disease/therapeutic intervention, are described without matching controls.

Level 5   Includes expert opinion where an opinion is based not on evidence but on 'first principles' (eg physiological or anatomical) or bench research.

GRADES OF RECOMMENDATION

Grade A   Usually depends on consistent level 1 evidence, and often means that the recommendation is effectively mandatory and placed within a clinical care pathway.

Grade B   Usually depends on consistent level 2 and/or 3 studies, or 'majority evidence' from RCTs.

Grade C   Usually depends on level 4 studies or 'majority evidence' from level 2/3 studies.

Grade D Usually given when the evidence is inconsistent/inconclusive or non-existent from studies that may vary in type from RCTs to case studies, or for expert opinion delivered without any analytical process.

Reference

1 Oxford Centre for Evidence-Based Medicine. *Levels of Evidence and Grades of Recommendations.* http://minerva.minervation.com/cebm/docs/levels.html

Practice guidance

1	*Access to services*
2	*Toilets and toileting*
3	*Prevention of bowel problems in old age*
4	*Identifying constipation in older people*
5	*Identifying risk factors for constipation in older people*
6	*Identifying faecal incontinence in older people*
7	*Identifying reversible risk factors and causes in older people with faecal incontinence*
8	*Assessment of faecal incontinence and constipation*
9	*Management of faecal incontinence and constipation*
10	*Laxatives in the management of constipation*
11	*Suggested elements of a bowel management programme in nursing and residential care homes*
12	*Psychological approaches to bowel care in dementia*

(*Strength of recommendation* [A]–[D]; see Appendix 1)

1. Access to services

▪ There should be access to a member of the primary healthcare team with the necessary skills to assess an older person with bowel difficulty and institute an appropriate initial regimen [D].

▪ Access to secondary or tertiary care should be along a well defined pathway of care to specialists with the appropriate knowledge, skills and attitudes to manage the problem effectively [C].

▪ A specialist continence advisory service should be available to all older people with bowel difficulty [B].

▪ Specialist training in continence promotion and bowel management should be available for all nurses involved in the care of older people [D].

2. Toilets and toileting

▪ A multidisciplinary assessment should be made of the older person's ability to access and use the toilet [D].

▪ The older person should be given the opportunity to use the toilet (either directly or by using a sani-chair or shower chair) rather than a bedside commode.

▪ Institutional/residential settings should have sani-chairs or shower chairs as well as commodes for residents' use [C].

▪ Toileting opportunities should be determined to suit individual needs and to maximise successful defaecation (eg after meals, after exercise/ mobilising) [D].

▪ Bedpans should be avoided for defaecation purposes [D].

▪ Commodes/sani-chairs/shower chairs should be in good condition (free from rust, rips and squeaky wheels) [D].

▪ Toilets/commodes/sani-chairs/shower chairs should provide a safe seated position for prolonged use by elderly people with skin vulnerability and trunk support problems (eg padded seat, back and arms, grab rails etc) [C].

▪ The person's bottom should never be visible to others, and transportation to the toilet and use of the toilet or commode should be carried out with due regard to privacy and dignity [D].

▪ The person should be given a direct method of calling for assistance when left on the toilet/commode [D].

▪ Methods to reduce noise and odour should be offered, particularly if the person is using a commode [D].

▪ If the patient has a commode in their living area that cannot be emptied immediately, a chemical toilet should be offered instead [C].

▪ Methods to facilitate bottom wiping should be available [D].

3. Prevention of bowel problems in old age

▪ Awareness of an older person's bowel habit should be seen as an essential part of their management or care plan [C].

▪ Obstetric care (particularly in the second stage of labour) and surgical management of anorectal disorders may have a role in prevention of later problems. For example, anorectal surgical procedures should be performed only by a trained coloproctology surgeon with special interest in pelvic floor abnormalities, and anal stretch procedures should no longer be carried out in adults [C].

▪ Prevention or prompt treatment of diarrhoea, particularly due to *Clostridium difficile* and similar infections in hospital and care settings, may help prevent consequent incontinence from developing [D].

▪ Strict antibiotic policies and handwashing by all staff before and after contact with patients should be employed to reduce the risk of infectious disease [B].

▪ Proactive planning and bowel management are needed in patients with problems known to have a high association with bowel problems (see Chapter 3) [B].

4. Identifying constipation in older people

▪ Self-reported constipation should be noted and specific symptoms should be routinely enquired about in all people aged 65 years and over in view of the high prevalence of the condition in this population [B].

▪ Both men and women in their eighth decade and beyond should be regularly screened for constipation problems as the prevalence increases with advancing age [B].

▪ A clear understanding of the specific bowel symptoms experienced by each older individual when reporting constipation is important in guiding the healthcare provider towards appropriate management of this common complaint [B].

▪ Reduced bowel movement frequency is not a sensitive clinical indicator for constipation in older people [B], though it is specific [C]. Difficulty with evacuation and rectal outlet delay should be carefully identified as these are primary symptoms in older individuals [B].

∎ A careful and objective assessment should be undertaken in all frail older individuals self-reporting constipation and/or difficulty with evacuation as these patients are at increased risk of clinical constipation and associated complications [B].

∎ Periodic objective assessment for constipation in elderly nursing home residents should be incorporated into routine nursing and medical care [B]. Patients unable to report symptoms due to cognitive or communication difficulties should be targeted [D]. Assessment should occur at a minimum every three months (three-monthly incidence rate of new-onset constipation is 7% in nursing home residents) and optimally monthly [C].

∎ All elderly people prescribed laxatives on a daily basis should be regularly reviewed for symptoms of constipation and the appropriateness of long-term laxative therapy [C].

∎ Constipation may be self-induced by reluctance to use institutional toilet facilities if these are not acceptable [C].

5. Identifying risk factors for constipation in older people

∎ The identification of risk factors for constipation in elderly individuals is critical to achieving effective management of the condition [B].

∎ A systematic process for identifying numerous risk factors in frail older people with constipation should be incorporated into good practice guidelines in primary care, acute hospitals and nursing homes [C].

∎ An integrative approach to risk assessment in constipated patients in all healthcare settings involving nursing and medical staff should be established [D].

∎ The following categories of patients are at increased risk of constipation and should be periodically and objectively assessed for the condition:
  – those taking more than five prescribed medications [B]
  – those taking anticholinergic drugs [B], opiates [B], iron [C], nifedipine/verapamil [B] or non-steroidal anti-inflammatory drugs [B]
  – non-ambulant individuals [B]
  – nursing home residents [B]
  – patients with Parkinson's disease [B], diabetes mellitus [B], spinal cord disease or injury [B], stroke [D]
  – patients with clinical dehydration [B]
  – patients with dementia [B] or depression [C]
  – patients with hypothyroidism, uraemia, hypokalaemia or hypercalcaemia [B].

6. Identifying faecal incontinence in older people

▪ Bowel continence status should be established by direct questioning and/or direct observation in:
  - nursing and residential home residents [B]
  - hospital inpatients aged 65 and over [C]
  - people aged 80 and over living at home [B]
  - older adults with impaired mobility [B]
  - older adults with impaired cognition [B]
  - older adults with neurological disease [B].

▪ General practitioners (GPs), primary care nurses, hospital ward staff, and long-term care staff should routinely enquire about bowel incontinence in frail older patients [B].

▪ Faecal incontinence case-finding should also include an assessment of how the patient (and carer where relevant) perceives the problem, for example, impact of symptoms on routine and social activities, 'how much does it bother you?' [D].

▪ Older patients with restricted ability to access primary care, such as nursing home residents and those with mobility and/or cognitive impairments, should be especially targeted for bowel continence screening [D].

▪ There are significant geographic variations in provision of specialist expertise in bowel care (both medical and nursing) which may affect case-finding in the community and in nursing homes [D].

▪ Education of healthcare providers with regard to raising awareness of the problem, plus methods of identification, assessment and management of faecal incontinence in older people, should be broad-ranging and include geriatricians, GPs, hospital physicians, hospital, community, general practice and long-term care nurses, and related disciplines (physiotherapists, occupational therapists, dieticians, pharmacists) [D].

▪ Continence nurse specialists should be trained in the management of faecal as well as urinary incontinence [D].

▪ Systematic outreach programmes should be implemented which make it easier for frail older people and those who care for them to volunteer the problem to their primary care provider [D]. Older people are likely to have similar misconceptions about faecal incontinence as urinary incontinence which inhibit them from reporting the symptom (ie that it is either a condition of ageing about which nothing can be done or not a problem to bother the doctor about).

7. Identifying reversible risk factors and causes in older people with faecal incontinence

∎ The following potentially modifiable risk factors for faecal incontinence should be carefully identified in all cases:

– constipation causing impaction and overflow [B]
– impaired mobility [B]
– diarrhoea or loose stools (eg laxative excess, drug-induced, dietary-related, infective) [B]
– neurological disease (eg Parkinson's disease [B], resolving stroke [C], diabetic-related autonomic neuropathy [B])
– delirium (as a reversible cause of cognitive impairment) [D]
– acute functional impairment [C]
– anal sphincter weakness [B]
– impaired vision and/or manual dexterity [D]
– problematic toilet access [D].

∎ All older people with faecal incontinence should be further assessed for reversible causes, regardless of their institutionalisation status [B].

∎ All frail older people with overflow incontinence should be assessed for potentially modifiable causes of constipation [B].

∎ Functional problems causing faecal incontinence should be identified early in the assessment of a frail older person [B].

∎ The symptom of loose stools should be elicited in all older people with any degree of faecal incontinence, and underlying causes rigorously sought [B].

∎ Colorectal carcinoma may present with the symptom of loose stools, and should be excluded where there is a marked change in bowel habit or other indicators (rectal bleeding, abdominal pain, weight loss, anaemia) [B].

∎ A standardised assessment of faecal incontinence in frail older people is required to ensure proper identification of underlying causes. Current difficulties relating to this are:

– Physicians do not prioritise assessment of faecal incontinence of frail older people (especially in nursing homes) [B]. Nurses may be more aware of the problem but are not always trained to look for underlying causes.
– Currently, few hospital wards, primary care practices or long-term care institutions have appropriate multidisciplinary protocols of case-finding and risk assessment.
– Nurses are not routinely trained to perform rectal examinations to evaluate stool retention.

▪ New ventures should be considered, for example multidisciplinary management of faecal incontinence in older people in intermediate and community care centres. The effectiveness of care pathways in assessing bowel problems in older people is presently unknown, but this approach should be explored as a nurse-led initiative.

8. Assessment of faecal incontinence and constipation

▪ Patients should have a multidisciplinary and multidimensional assessment prior to planning care. Suggested components of the history are detailed in Chapter 4 [D].

▪ Physical examination should include [D]:
  – abdominal examination for presence of palpable faecal mass(es)
  – anal inspection for evidence of soiling, rectal prolapse, peri-anal scarring, gaping anus and/or perineal descent
  – digital anal examination to assess anal resting tone and squeeze
  – digital rectal examination to determine whether there are abnormal rectal lesions or faecal loading of the rectum; if the rectum is loaded, stool consistency should be assessed.
  – cognitive assessment
  – toileting skills and toilet facilities.

▪ Investigations may be indicated as follows:
  – *Abdominal radiograph*: an empty rectum does not always exclude the diagnosis of constipation. In this situation, an abdominal radiograph may help to determine whether faecal loading is present and to assess its extent. It may also be useful when evaluating the degree of bowel obstruction secondary to faecal impaction, to rule out acute complications of impaction such as sigmoid volvulus and stercoral perforation and to identify colonic dysmotility [D].
  – *Anorectal physiology tests*, including anal manometry, endo-anal ultrasound, external sphincter electromyography and defaecating proctography, are not usually required in the frail elderly as, even in surgical clinics, they tend not to alter the clinical examination conclusions or the management plan [D].
  – *Investigation of symptoms* of constipation, diarrhoea and/or faecal incontinence may be required to exclude significant bowel pathology because any one of them can be the presenting symptom of colonic disease [C].
  – Colonoscopy or barium enema may be indicated, but bowel preparation may cause acute diarrhoea [C].

9. Management of faecal incontinence and constipation

▪ There is no evidence on patient-based outcomes for management.
▪ Multiple interventions are often required to maintain normal bowel function. Approaches to management include:
  – determination and utilisation of the individual's premorbid bowel pattern [D]
  – bowel retraining [C]
  – non-pharmacological approaches, such as exercise, abdominal massage, timing of meals, coffee and other caffeine intake [C]
  – rectal evacuants used in a hierarchy: glycerine suppository, bisacodyl suppository, micro-enema, phosphate enema [D]
  – digital stimulation may initiate defaecation for some patients [D]
  – rectal washouts can be used in the place of suppositories – tap water or saline may be used
  – metabolic monitoring is important [D]
  – manual evacuation: other methods of bowel evacuation are preferred, but planned manual evacuation on a regular basis is an acceptable method of bowel management in frail older people if other alternatives are unsuccessful [D]
  – oestrogen replacement should be considered in selected patients [C]
  – patients with faecal incontinence who are able to comply should be taught anal sphincter exercises; these should be taught by digital rectal examination or biofeedback, as many patients practise incorrectly [C].
  – the role of electrical stimulation is not established
  – *surgery*: full thickness rectal prolapse will usually require surgical intervention in frail older people using a transanal approach [C]. Sphincter repair and stoma formation should not be ruled out in this group, but decisions require careful consideration with the quality of life of both the individual and the carer as the primary concern [D].
  – *containment*: there are no good answers to containing faecal incontinence. The anal plug may be suitable in a minority of cases. Scrupulous skin care and attention to odour control are essential [D].

10. Laxatives in the management of constipation

▪ Exclude an organic cause for the constipation [A].

▪ Faecal impaction should be resolved using strong osmotic laxatives and phosphate enemas. Occasionally, disimpaction under anaesthetic may be required [A].

▪ Patients with idiopathic constipation require initial conservative therapy:
  − attention to diet [B]
  − adequate fluid intake [C]
  − adequate fibre intake [B]
  − optimisation of neurological function and mobility [C]
  − instruction about toileting behaviour [C]
  − coexisting illness and medications exacerbating bowel function should be sought and corrected [B].

▪ In patients unresponsive to conservative measures:
  − consider laxatives [A]
  − consider bulking laxatives if fluid and fibre intake is suboptimal [B]
  − if additional treatment is required, combined bulking and stimulant laxatives are advised (stimulant laxatives on their own can be associated with a significant incidence of side effects) [B]
  − if patients remain symptomatic, an osmotic laxative may be used; cheaper laxatives (magnesium sulphate or magnesium hydroxide) are as effective as more expensive alternatives such as lactulose and lactitol [B]
  − enemas or suppositories may be required in addition to laxative therapy [C].

11. Suggested elements of a bowel management programme in nursing and residential care homes

▪ Enhance resident mobility.

▪ Ensure residents have sufficient fluids.

▪ Review medications that could cause bowel problems.

▪ Provide a diet high in fibre.

▪ Ensure residents have privacy and time to open bowels.

▪ Encourage residents to use the toilet after breakfast.

▪ Ensure availability of suitable toilet adaptations and alternatives to suit individual needs.

▪ Monitor bowel actions.

▪ Carry out a bowel assessment for all new residents and re-assess periodically.

12. Psychological approaches to bowel care in dementia

■ Local protocols should be adopted within primary and secondary care agencies to ensure specialist support and safeguards to enable good nursing practice [B].

■ Care plans should include:

– details of steps taken to establish a cause for abnormal bowel function [B]

– details of interventions carried out to improve bowel function [B]

– baseline information and objective measures of change [B].

■ Demonstrable competencies among nursing and care staff in the psychological care of patients with dementia should be developed and kept up to date [C].